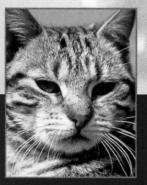
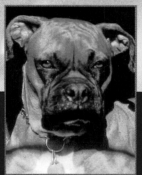
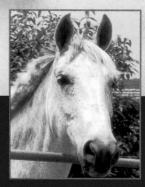
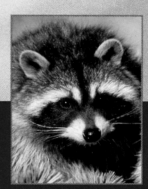
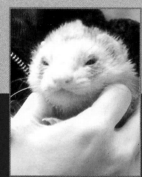

RABIES:
Guidelines for Medical Professionals

Library of Congress No. 99-95727
ISBN 1-884254-47-0

The opinions expressed in this publication are those of the authors and do not
necessarily reflect the opinions of the publisher or the sponsor.

Designed and Published by Veterinary Learning Systems
275 Phillips Blvd.
Trenton, NJ 08618

Sponsored by an educational grant from Merial

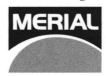

Contents

Participants

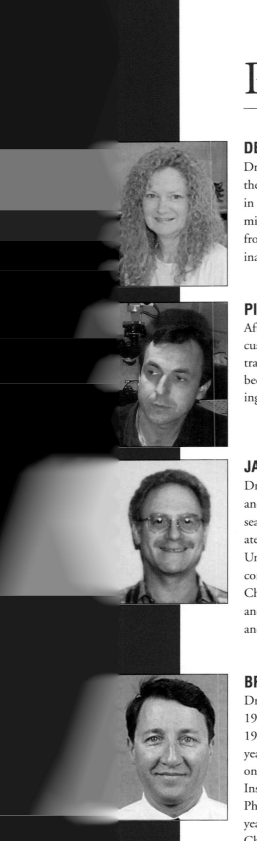

DEBORAH J. BRIGGS, PhD

Dr. Briggs received her PhD from Kansas State University in 1989 and was named Director of the Rabies Laboratory at Kansas State University in 1990. She was promoted to Full Professor in 1998. Dr. Briggs has been the Chair of the United States Animal Health Association Committee for Rabies since 1994. Dr. Briggs recently received the Guide Dog Access Partners Award from Guide Dog Users Inc. for her role in helping blind people gain access to Hawaii by eliminating the quarantine restrictions for their guide dogs.

PIERRE-EMMANUEL CECCALDI, PhD

After receiving his PhD in Neuroscience in 1989 at the Université Paris VI, where his work focused on the axonal transport of the rabies virus, Dr. Ceccaldi spent 2 years in postdoctoral training on the control of neurotransmitter release at the University of Milan in Italy. He has been a Research Assistant at the Rabies Unit of the Pasteur Institute in Paris since 1993, studying the mechanisms of rabies pathogenesis.

JAMES E. CHILDS, ScD

Dr. Childs received his doctoral degree from The Johns Hopkins University School of Hygiene and Public Health in 1982. After postdoctoral research at the United States Army Medical Research Institute for Infectious Diseases, he held the positions of Assistant Professor and Associate Professor in the Department of Immunology and Infectious Diseases at The Johns Hopkins University. He joined the Centers for Disease Control and Prevention in 1992, where he has continued his research on viral and rickettsial zoonoses. He is currently Epidemiology Section Chief and Acting Branch Chief in the Viral and Rickettsial Zoonoses Branch, Division of Viral and Rickettsial Diseases, National Center for Infectious Diseases, Centers for Disease Control and Prevention, in Atlanta.

BRUNO B. CHOMEL, DVM, PhD

Dr. Chomel received his DVM in 1978 from the Lyon Veterinary School in Lyon, France. In 1979 he became a faculty member of the Lyon Veterinary School, where he remained until 1990, becoming Professor and Chair of the Infectious Diseases Department in 1989, the same year he received his "Habilitation à Diriger la Recherche," or Research Director degree. While on the faculty at the Veterinary School, he received his MS in Microbiology from the Pasteur Institute in Paris (1981), his MS in Immunology from the University of Lyon (1982), and his PhD in Microbiology from Claude Bernard University in Lyon (1984). He also served for 2 years as an Epidemic Intelligence Service Officer for the Centers for Disease Control. Dr. Chomel joined the faculty of the School of Veterinary Medicine at the University of California, Davis, in 1990, becoming Professor of Zoonoses. His research centers on cat-scratch disease and *Bartonella* infections in domestic animals and wildlife and on the epidemiology of rabies and plague. He is also Director of the World Health Organization/Pan American Health Organization (WHO/PAHO) Collaborating Center on New and Emerging Zoonoses at UC-Davis.

DAVID W. DREESEN, DVM, MPVM
Diplomate ACVPM

Dr. Dreesen has been involved in rabies control, epidemiologic studies, and human and animal vaccine trials since 1967, through his professional positions as State Public Health Veterinarian with the Georgia Department of Human Resources, Scientist with the Pan American Health Organization, and more than 21 years as Professor with the College of Veterinary Medicine at the University of Georgia. Dr. Dreesen retired from the University in July 1998 and now owns a private consulting business specializing in rabies as well as food-borne diseases. He is a member of the AVMA and is a Diplomate in the American College of Veterinary Preventive Medicine (ACVPM), as well as a Charter Diplomate in the Epidemiology Specialty of the ACVPM. Dr. Dreesen has worked on rabies projects and has lectured on rabies in more than 17 countries throughout the world.

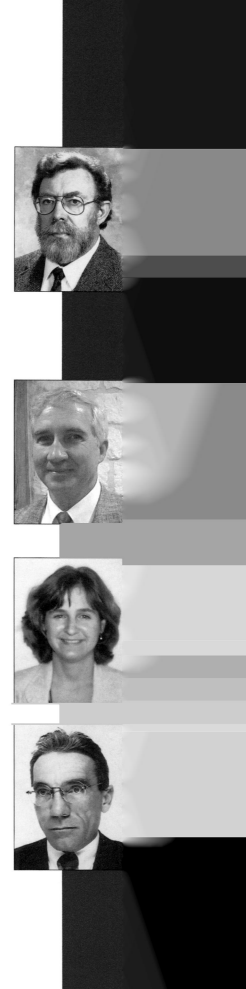

GAYNE FEARNEYHOUGH, BS, DVM

Dr. Fearneyhough completed his DVM degree at Texas A&M University in 1976. Upon graduation, he entered private veterinary practice in San Antonio. In 1978 Dr. Fearneyhough became a staff member of an emergency care veterinary practice in Houston before opening his own clinic in the Houston suburb of Missouri City. He became Zoonosis Control Regional Veterinarian for the Texas Department of Health in Tyler, Texas, in 1992, responsible for the surveillance, monitoring, and reporting of zoonotic diseases such as rabies, arbovirus encephalitis, Rocky Mountain spotted fever, and Lyme disease in East Texas. In 1993 he became Program Director of the Oral Rabies Vaccination Program for the Texas Department of Health, a program developed to contain and eventually eliminate the canine strain of rabies from Texas.

JENNIFER H. McQUISTON, DVM, MS

Dr. McQuiston received her DVM in 1997 and her MS in Molecular Biology in 1998 from Virginia-Maryland Regional College of Veterinary Medicine, Virginia Polytechnic Institute and State University. Her research interests have focused on the epidemiology of viral and rickettsial diseases. Currently, she is an Epidemic Intelligence Service Officer assigned to the Viral and Rickettsial Zoonoses Branch, Division of Viral and Rickettsial Diseases, National Center for Infectious Diseases, Centers for Disease Control and Prevention, in Atlanta.

F.-X. MESLIN, DVM

After receiving his DVM in 1981 from Claude Bernard University in Lyon, France, Dr. Meslin completed postgraduate training in Food Hygiene and Inspection at the Institute of Tropical Veterinary Medicine in Maisons-Alfort, France. His 15-year association with the World Health Organization began in 1984, when he served as Coordinator of the Veterinary Public Health Unit Project for Human and Canine Rabies Control in Developing Countries for the Division of Communicable Diseases. He became Secretary of the Mediterranean Zoonoses Control Programme in 1987. By 1992, he had become Chief of the Veterinary Public Health Unit. In 1995, he became Team Leader of Zoonotic Diseases in the Division of Emerging and Other Communicable Diseases Surveillance and Control; he became Chief of Zoonotic Diseases in 1998. He is currently Team Coordinator of Animal and Food-Related Public Health Risks for the Department of Communicable Diseases Surveillance and Response.

(continued)

Participants *(continued)*

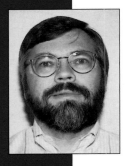

CHARLES EDWARD RUPPRECHT, VMD, MS, PhD

Dr. Rupprecht received his MS in Zoology from the University of Wisconsin (1980), his VMD from the School of Veterinary Medicine at the University of Pennsylvania (1985), and his PhD in Biology from the University of Wisconsin (1986). Between 1982 and 1992 he was employed in the Rabies Section of the Wistar Institute of Anatomy and Biology in Philadelphia before moving to the Center for Neurovirology at Thomas Jefferson University in Philadelphia. He joined the Centers for Disease Control and Prevention in 1993, serving as Chief of the Rabies Section and Director of the World Health Organization Collaborating Center for Reference and Research on Rabies. Over the past 20 years, he has authored or coauthored more than 100 published communications on rabies diagnosis, pathogenesis, epidemiology, prevention, and control.

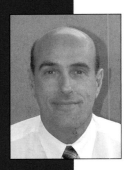

CHARLES V. TRIMARCHI, MS

Mr. Trimarchi received his BS degree from the State University of New York at Albany in 1968 and his MS from Union College in Schenectady in 1982. He joined the Rabies Laboratory at the New York State Department of Health's Wadsworth Center Laboratories in 1968, serving as Director since 1979. His research interests have been the development and evaluation of improved rabies diagnostic methods and the investigation of the natural history of bat rabies. He serves as Chairman of the New York State Interdepartmental Rabies Committee and as Technical Advisor to the National Association of State Public Health Veterinarians, Animal Rabies Control Committee.

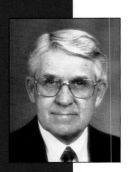

KENT R. VAN KAMPEN, DVM, PhD
Diplomate ACVP

After earning his DVM from Colorado State University in 1964 and his PhD from the University of California, Davis, in 1967, Dr. Van Kampen became a research pathologist with the U.S. Department of Agriculture. He later cofounded Intermountain Laboratories, Inc., and served as its General Manager and Vice President of Research. In 1976 Dr. Van Kampen became the Chairman of the Department of Animal, Dairy, and Veterinary Sciences at Utah State University. He later served in a variety of executive positions with several biotechnical companies. In 1993 he organized The Van Kampen Group, Inc., a professional consulting group that provides assistance to medical industries in the fields of pathology, regulatory affairs, clinical studies, and business management.

Introduction

The purpose of this publication is to provide public health officials, veterinarians, and other human and animal health professionals with a rabies resource guide covering several current topics of interest.

The scope of coverage encompasses a global review of both human and animal rabies as it relates to pathogenesis, clinical disease, and diagnosis of rabies in humans, domesticated mammals, and mammals that serve as wildlife reservoirs. Effective postexposure prophylaxis (treatment) programs are also detailed.

Various sections provide information on preventive immunization programs (preexposure immunoprophylaxis) utilizing conventional as well as innovative new vaccines that are available for humans, domestic animals, and wild animals. Some of these immunization programs, along with highly variable quarantine laws, have a direct impact on the movement of companion animals from country to country.

Of special interest to readers is the continuously high number of rabies-induced human deaths, despite tremendous advances in the effectiveness and availability of vaccines and postexposure treatment over the past several years. Expense estimates associated with rabies prevention and especially postexposure treatment will likely exceed most expectations.

A special "thank you" goes out to all of the authors and to Dr. Miguel Escobar for their extra effort in making this publication possible. The authors of each section have had the freedom to express their views as they have deemed appropriate.

We hope you will find this guide a useful supplement to your "rabies library."

Don Hildebrand
Vice President
Merial

Foreword

Charles Edward Rupprecht, VMD, MS, PhD
Chief, Rabies Section
Centers for Disease Control and Prevention, Atlanta, Georgia

Rabies presents a unique challenge to today's thinking biomedical professional, particularly because of its historic dread, prevalent mythos, and paradoxical nature. Although it is an acute, progressive, viral encephalitis transmitted via the bite of infected animals and possesses the highest case fatality of any agent once clinical signs develop, it is almost always preventable if exposure has been recognized and prompt and proper modern prophylaxis can be initiated. This infectious disease hails from antiquity, but new aspects concerning its basic causation and epizootiology await discovery. The etiologic agents, assigned to the family Rhabdoviridae, genus *Lyssavirus*, reside on all inhabited continents and contain at least seven putative genotypes, only one of which, rabies virus, occurs in the New World. Birds can be infected under experimental conditions, yet mammals are the only defined natural hosts. All mammals are believed to be susceptible to infection, but reservoirs are confined solely to Carnivora and Chiroptera. Both genetic sequence and antigenic data clearly demonstrate that, although once believed to be a single entity, rabies is caused by highly compartmentalized, dynamic virus variants that persist among many different hosts. The dog is the single prominent global reservoir, particularly in developing countries, while in North America these taxa include arctic, red, and gray foxes, coyotes, skunks, raccoons, mongooses, and bats. Neither current experimental nor epidemiologic data support the widespread concept of a true "carrier state," but the incubation period (when the virus is noninfectious) is extremely variable, ranging from days to years. Lyssaviruses may attain the title of penultimate neurotropic, neuroinvasive, and neurovirulent agents; nevertheless, they defy simple detection until they reach the nervous system, through as yet inexplicable processes. Rapt in the collective consciousness with stereotypical maniacal presentation, these obligate parasites outwit clinicians continually because signs of illness may be quite subtle, and the only truly pathognomonic syndrome may relate to a presentation uncharacteristic of the norm. Often subjectively labeled as defective in basic strategy because of catastrophic outcome, in another perspective the host is merely excess baggage as these viruses effect their own transmission to a new residence by surreptitious behavioral alteration before the final curtain call. As rabies is believed to be controlled in one arena, it becomes entrenched, emerges, and reemerges in another. Numerous recent examples demonstrate that the purposeful or accidental translocation of infected wildlife has led to the invasion of unoccupied niches, some with dramatic consequences. Because of the ample public health, agricultural, and conservational threats posed by the local, regional, and international movement of infected animals, many diverse professionals have a primary responsibility in the surveillance, diagnosis, prevention, and control of this disease in order to minimize the opportunity for an unrecognized biologic oddity to emerge as tomorrow's outbreak. What will the new millennium have in store for this quintessential zoonotic horror? A cure—or vaccine-resistant variants? Significant strides toward dog rabies elimination—or the emergence of ever more vagile hosts? Development of better, less expensive, even edible, biologics—or even further disparity between the "haves" and the "have nots?" One thing is certain: The continuing education provided by *Rabies: Guidelines for Medical Professionals*, written by some of the top authorities in the field, should remain a key ingredient in the coming storm, providing ample rationale to resist assuming a cavalier attitude toward a bug with an inherent biotic capacity to return with a vengeance.

Global Review of Human and Animal Rabies

F.-X. Meslin, DVM
Team Coordinator, Animal and Food-Related Public Health Risks
Department of Communicable Diseases Surveillance and Response
World Health Organization
Geneva, Switzerland

RABIES IS WIDELY DISTRIBUTED THROUGHOUT THE WORLD AND IS PRESENT IN ALL CONTINENTS BUT AUSTRALIA. THE NUMBER AND SIZE OF RABIES-FREE COUNTRIES, TERRITORIES, OR AREAS ARE SMALL COMPARED TO THOSE OF RABIES-AFFECTED AREAS. ACCORDING TO THE WORLD SURVEY OF RABIES FOR 1996, 46 OUT OF 153 COUNTRIES AND TERRITORIES REPORTED NO RABIES FOR THAT YEAR AND HAD NO RABIES IN 1995. MANY RABIES-FREE COUNTRIES AND TERRITORIES ARE ISLANDS OF THE DEVELOPED WORLD (E.G., AUSTRALIA, JAPAN, NEW ZEALAND, UNITED KINGDOM) AND THE DEVELOPING WORLD (E.G., BARBADOS, FIJI, MALDIVES, AND SEYCHELLES). IN ADDITION, PARTS OF NORTHERN AND SOUTHERN CONTINENTAL EUROPE (E.G., SCANDINAVIAN COUNTRIES, SPAIN, PORTUGAL, GREECE) AND LATIN AMERICA (E.G., URUGUAY AND CHILE) ARE ALSO FREE OF RABIES.

A large number of mammalian animal species are involved throughout the world in rabies maintenance and transmission. Many reservoirs of rabies are terrestrial species, mainly wild carnivora, for example, coyotes, red, arctic, and gray foxes, jackals, mongooses, raccoons, skunks, and wolves. Most important additions to this list are privately owned, community-owned, and ownerless, sometimes feral dogs that remain the main reservoir and transmitter of rabies to humans in developing countries. Many other animal species are susceptible but do not transmit the disease further: They are victims of rabies and usually epidemiologic dead-ends. Many animal victims are production or draft animals (e.g., cattle, camels, and horses), and their deaths add to the economic burden represented by the disease. In addition, many bat species are hosts, transmitters, or victims of rabies. For example, bat rabies is reported in the United States, certain Latin American countries, some European countries, parts of Africa, and, more recently, Australia.

In most countries, only one terrestrial animal species maintains rabies in nature (e.g., the red fox in western Europe, the dog in most developing countries). In certain countries, however, different and independent transmission cycles exist in several terrestrial reservoir species (e.g., skunk, raccoon, coyote, and gray fox in the United States, mongoose, dog, bat-eared fox, and jackal in South Africa, dog and wolf in Iran, dog and fox in Israel). Furthermore, as observed in some countries where only dog rabies was previously reported, wildlife rabies may emerge when the incidence

Worldwide, it is estimated that between 45,000 and 60,000 persons die of rabies each year.

The views expressed in this article are solely the responsibility of the author.

of dog rabies is drastically reduced or the disease is eliminated in dogs (e.g., South Korea).

Worldwide, it is estimated that between 45,000 and 60,000 persons die of rabies each year. Most of these deaths (40,000 to 50,000) occur in Asian countries: India officially reports 30,000 deaths and Bangladesh, 2,000. In Pakistan estimates range from 2,000 to 6,000 deaths annually. In addition, some 50 million doses of vaccines are used in 10 million human postexposure treatments worldwide. About 8 million of them are applied in developing countries. The number of postexposure treatments in humans varies greatly from country to country. In developing countries, vaccine cost is the main factor affecting the number of postexposure treatments applied; availability outside major urban centers is the second important factor. In some developing countries where rabies is endemic to most parts of the national territory, as many as 300 to 400 persons are treated per 100,000 inhabitants, while in other developing countries, fewer than 40 treatments are provided. Costs of modern, safe, and potent human rabies vaccine represent the major component (e.g., 30% in Thailand) of the total economic burden represented by rabies.

Besides prophylactic vaccination of humans, many dogs throughout the world receive rabies shots. It is estimated that at least 50 million dogs are vaccinated each year against rabies either in private practices or during national campaigns organized by ministries of health or agriculture. In many parts of Asia and Africa, the vaccination coverage established in the dog population (30% to 50%) is not high enough to break the transmission cycle of the disease.

Sharp declines have been reported in the number of human deaths in two Asian countries (China and Thailand) and in many Latin American countries, where only 118 deaths were reported in 1997, thanks to the regional urban rabies control program initiated in 1986. In China and Thailand the number of human rabies deaths decreased by about 90% within 15 to 20 years—the factors for this improvement are certainly manifold. It seems clear, however, that in both countries an improved postexposure treatment and a vaccine delivery system with a major shift in the type of vaccine produced, from brain tissue–based toward cell culture–based products, played a major role. On the other hand, the trend toward a decline in the number of cases in animals has been reported in many European countries. In 10 of these countries a 95% reduction in the number of cases in animals, mainly foxes, was reported over the past 9 years. This decrease followed the massive use of the oral immunization technique for foxes and the dispersal over wide areas of more than 90 million vaccine baits since 1989. Remarkable decreases have also been noted in Texas (United States) and in Canada, where oral vaccination projects targeting coyotes and foxes, respectively, have been conducted. Still, trends showing an increase have been reported recently in some parts of the world such as certain eastern African countries (e.g., Mozambique and Madagascar), some new independent states (e.g., Kazakhstan), and some Asian countries (e.g., Pakistan and Sri Lanka) where dog rabies prevails.

Control of rabies is carried out with different levels of intensity in both developing and developed countries. In many countries in which the dog is the reservoir of the virus, few activities are underway to prevent rabies occurrence in humans and to control rabies in dogs, even when the number of human deaths is high. This is the case in, for example, Bangladesh, Cambodia, Laos, Nepal, and Pakistan in Asia, as well as most African, east Mediterranean, and Arabic peninsular countries. On the other hand, some countries report having improved their postexposure treatment delivery systems in conjunction with significant activities for dog rabies control. In some countries these activities have led to a sustainable reduction in dog rabies as previously reported for China and Thailand, as well as South Africa, Iran, and most Latin American countries. In other countries (e.g., Morocco, Tunisia, and Sri Lanka) these activities have led to containment of the rabies situation. In some countries where wildlife-mediated rabies prevails, programs for the oral vaccination of wildlife reservoirs for which vaccines have been shown to be safe and effective are underway. These actions are conducted on a large-scale basis in western Europe and also in Texas. Smaller scale oral vaccination projects are underway in Ontario (Canada) for foxes, in certain states in the United States for raccoons, and in more and more central and eastern European countries.

In conclusion, it should be borne in mind that most human rabies cases reported worldwide follow exposure to rabid dogs and are reported in developing countries, mainly in Asia. Remarkable decreases in the incidence of rabies in humans and animals have been reported recently in both developing and developed countries. Failure in adequately tackling the problem is also reported in many developing countries where rabies represents a serious public health burden. As a consequence, millions of dollars are spent annually in many countries in an attempt to prevent and control rabies in humans and animals (mainly dogs), but without progress. These expenses, currently estimated (in U.S. dollars) at $500 million a year in developing countries alone, are likely to further increase if no comprehensive plans for disease control and elimination in animal reservoirs are undertaken.

Most human rabies cases reported worldwide follow exposure to rabid dogs and are reported in developing countries, mainly in Asia.

The Pathogenesis of Rabies

Pierre-Emmanuel Ceccaldi, PhD
Research Assistant, Rabies Unit, Pasteur Institute, Paris, France

Rabies virus, a member of the *Lyssavirus* genus, is a neurotropic agent that causes an acute central nervous system (CNS) disease in all mammals, leading almost always to death. Although the disease of rabies has been known since antiquity and the first prophylactic vaccinal treatment was established by Pasteur 100 years ago, the visualization of the rabies virus by electron microscopy was not accomplished until 1962 by Matsumoto.[1] Rabies virions are on average 180 nm long and 75 nm wide bullet-shaped cylinders (Figure 1). They are surrounded by a lipid bilayer envelope from the membrane of the infected cell. The membrane provides anchorage for the trimers of glycoprotein (G protein) that cover the outer surface of the particle. The M protein is located on the inner surface of the viral envelope, where it interacts with both the cytoplasmic tail of the G protein and the helical nucleocapsid; the latter contains the negative single-stranded RNA genome (11,932 nucleotides) and is tightly embedded with nucleoprotein (N protein), phosphoprotein (NS protein), and polymerase (L protein). Although in the past decades great progress has been made with respect to the molecular biology of the rabies virus,[2] the majority of the mechanisms of rabies pathogenesis are still not fully understood.

EARLY STEPS OF INFECTION

Rabies virus is transmitted mainly by bite-inflicted deposition of rabies virus–laden saliva or contamination of scratch wounds, although natural transmission through the mucosal membrane could occur.[3,4] Natural transmission, much less frequent than bite transmission, occurs via consumption of frozen rabid carcasses (Arctic region) or via airborne transmission as reported in bat caves. Although neurotropism is a major feature associated with rabies infection, a crucial point in the early steps of rabies virus infection remains to be determined, that is, whether the virus enters peripheral nerves directly (before migration to the CNS) or whether it proceeds through an indirect mechanism after replication in tissues outside of the CNS.

Classic experiments indicate that the virus is able to leave the site within a few hours following inoculation.[4] Using a model of viral inoculation in the mouse masseter muscle, Shankar and associates[5] showed that viral RNA is detected in the trigeminal ganglia as early as 18 hours postinfection. This finding indicates that the time between inoculation and departure of virus

Whether the rabies virus enters peripheral nerves directly or whether it proceeds through an indirect mechanism after replication in tissues outside of the CNS remains to be determined.

12

from the inoculation site is not sufficient for replication and that rabies virus is able to invade the nerve directly, without prior replication in the muscle. However, using immunofluorescence and electron microscopy techniques, Murphy and colleagues[6] showed that myocytes at the site of inoculation are infected. Moreover, on a skunk model infected with a skunk street strain (i.e., field strain), it was shown that the muscle fibers at the site of inoculation can be directly infected by the viral inoculum.[7] Tsiang and coworkers[8–10] infected cultured myotubes from rat embryos with either fixed strain (i.e., laboratory strain) or street strain. They found that differentiated myocytes were susceptible to both strains, although only moderately, but that production of infectious virus was significantly enhanced in the street strain. This seems to indicate that the fox isolate street strain underwent an amplification step in the myocytes prior to the infection of peripheral nerve endings but that this amplification step did not occur in the fixed strain. This might make it possible for the rabies virus to persist locally for long periods at the site of inoculation and thus for naturally occurring rabies cases to develop after prolonged incubation periods.

Whichever are the first host cells to be infected by rabies virus, that is, myocytes or peripheral nerve cells, several studies have focused on the identification of the cellular receptor for the rabies virus, which could be recognized by the rabies glycoprotein. Some reports indicate that phospholipids, gangliosides, and carbohydrate moieties may be components of a complex receptor for the rabies virus.[10] A rather good candidate for a rabies virus receptor is the nicotinic acetylcholine receptor[11]; this assumption is based mainly on inhibition experiments with nicotinic cholinergic antagonists, immunofluorescence localization, overlay binding assays, and sequence homologies between the rabies glycoprotein and snake venom

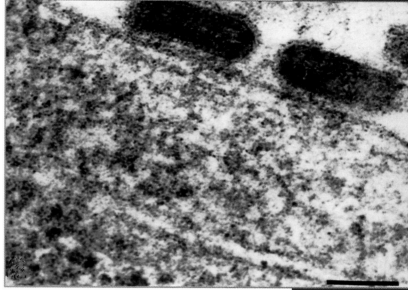

curaremimetic neurotoxins. However, the capacity of rabies virus to infect stretch proprioceptors, sensory endings, and some cell lines that do not express the acetylcholine receptor indicates that rabies virus can use other receptors; for example, the neural cell adhesion molecule has recently been identified as a putative receptor for rabies virus.[12] The subsequent step of viral infection, that is, virus penetration, has been shown to occur by either adsorptive endocytosis or direct fusion with the viral membrane. In as few as 5 minutes after infection, electron microscopy has allowed visualization of groups of virions within coated or uncoated vesicles.[13] Once these virions are present in the lysosomes, a pH-dependent conformational change allows the release of rabies nucleocapsid into the cytoplasm,[14] where transcription and replication can occur.[2]

SPREAD OF VIRUS WITHIN THE PERIPHERAL NERVOUS SYSTEM

After viral uptake at neuronal endings, virus is transported to the CNS in both sensory and motor fibers.[4,15] Axonal transport of rabies virus had been suggested earlier, because removal of perineural structures could not modify the viral spread to the CNS. Evidence of the axonal transport of rabies virus has been definitively given by

Figure 1—Electron micrograph of rabies virions in the vicinity of 7-day-old human dorsal root ganglia cultures. Cultures were performed as described in reference 18 and infected with a fixed rabies virus strain. (Scale bar = 100 nm.)

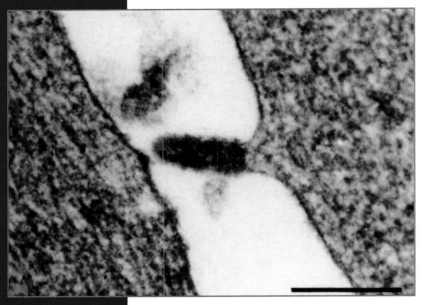

Figure 2—Electron micrograph of viral budding from a neuron of 7-day-old human dorsal root ganglia cultures. Cultures were performed as described in reference 18 and infected with a fixed rabies virus strain. (Scale bar = 200 nm.)

using colchicine and vinblastine; these two drugs, which inhibit the axonal transport via microtubule network disruption, can prevent rabies virus spread to the CNS.[16,17] In vitro, in sensory neurons from rat or human origin, both anterograde and retrograde axonal transports are efficient in transporting rabies virus.[18–20] In this system, the velocity of the retrograde axonal transport of rabies virus is in the range of 25 to 50 mm per day,[19] which can be classified as a fast axonal transport mechanism. This can be related to the value that has been calculated in vivo, where the spread of virus in the oculomotor and optic nerves through retrograde axonal transport is about 12 mm per day.[21] It is still not known in which state (membranous vacuole or nucleocapsid) the virus particle is transported.

SPREAD OF VIRUS WITHIN THE CENTRAL NERVOUS SYSTEM

Once it has reached the CNS, rabies replication takes place primarily in the neurons, and the viral spread has been shown to occur in a transneuronal manner. Electron microscopy of the brain of infected animals has shown viral budding from the perikaryal and dendritic plasma membranes, including the postsynaptic membrane.[7] After viral budding (Figure 2) and

uptake by the adjacent axon terminal, the virion is transported via retrograde axonal transport to the dendrites and the cell body of the subsequent neuron. Retrograde axonal transport of the rabies virus has been demonstrated by stereotactic inoculation experiments in the rat brain.[22,23] This kind of transport seems to be predominant in the first steps of brain infection and allows the virus to infect almost all brain areas.[24] It is noteworthy that in natural rabies infection, a widespread distribution of rabies antigens is generally seen at the time of euthanasia or death (Figures 3 and 4), although in a few cases infection could be restricted to the spinal cord. It cannot be excluded that anterograde axonal transport could be used in addition to retrograde transport in viral spread,[20] although this would occur in later stages of infection. The release of intracellular virions through disruption of necrotic neurons does not seem to have a role in viral spread, because neuronal degeneration is not a major feature of rabies infection. In the same way, dissemination through the cerebrospinal fluid could occur but only in the late stages of infection.[25]

NEUROTROPISM

Neurotropism is a hallmark of rabies virus (Figures 5 and 6); some rabies virus strains have been reported to infect non-neuronal cells such as muscular cells,[8,9] lymphocytes, glial cells,[26] and cells of peripheral tissues outside of the CNS (see further discussion in references 4 and 24). However, the neurotropism of rabies virus is demonstrated by the means of viral spread (axonal transport), the high susceptibility of neurons to rabies infection,[10,27] the high potential of most neurons to yield high viral titers,[10] and, finally, the neural dysfunction induced by rabies infection (further discussion follows).

HISTOPATHOLOGY

No external abnormality is generally observed by macroscopic examination of the brain, except for a variable degree of cerebral edema.[26] Microscopic changes such as perivascular cuffing and neuronal necrosis are sparse compared to the extent of infection, which shows a widespread distribution when studied by fluorescent antibody technique. This technique demonstrates that most of the neurons throughout the brain can be infected; when searching for the pathognomonic histologic feature of rabies, that is, the Negri body (1–7 μm neuronal cytoplasmic eosinophilic inclusion), an underevaluation of the number of infected cells may occur, because this sign is inconsistent. Electron microscopy observations reveal that viral antigens are found within the Negri bodies (as well as in the so-called "lyssa bodies"), although viral antigens are not confined to these bodies.[26] Apoptosis has been shown to occur within the CNS of experimentally infected animals,[28] although its relevance in pathogenesis is still unclear. In fact, the most striking histopathologic changes are often seen in the spinal cord, where lymphocytic infiltration, neuronal degeneration of the anterior horn, and microglial cell proliferation are often seen, especially in the paralytic form of rabies.

Spongiform lesions of the CNS have been reported during natural rabies infection in animals such as skunk, fox, horse, cow, cat, and sheep[4,24]; these lesions are often localized in the thalamic nuclei and in the inner layers of the cerebral cortex. Such changes do not occur during experimental rabies infection of rodents.[24] Interestingly, the extent of membrane-bound vacuolization does not seem to correlate with the amount of viral antigen,[29] which means that these changes are due to an indirect effect of the infection, such as neurotransmitter imbalance in, for example, excitatory amino acids (aspartate and glutamate).

NEURAL DYSFUNCTION

The minimal cellular destruction during rabies infection rapidly led to the hypothesis that the clinical picture was due to neural

Figure 3—Rabies virus–infected cells in the cerebellum of a rat brain. Day 5 postinfection. Viral inclusions are visualized on cryostat sections with a fluorescein-isothiocyanate–labeled anti–rabies virus nucleocapsid polyclonal serum. (Scale bar = 30 μm.)

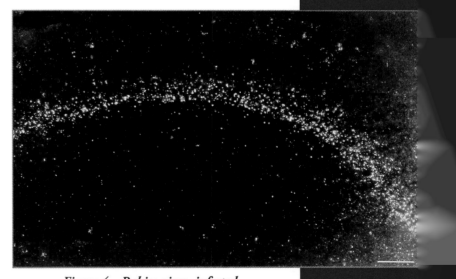

Figure 4—Rabies virus–infected cells in the hippocampal region of a rat brain. Day 5 postinfection. Viral inclusions are visualized on cryostat sections with a fluorescein-isothiocyanate–labeled anti–rabies virus nucleocapsid polyclonal serum. (Scale bar = 60 μm.)

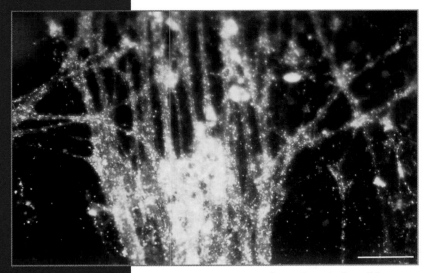

Figure 5—Rabies virus–infected human dorsal root ganglial neurons in culture. Day 3 postinfection. Viral inclusions are visualized with a fluorescein-isothiocyanate–labeled anti–rabies virus nucleocapsid polyclonal serum. Viral inclusions are present in the cell soma as well as in the neuritic extensions. (Scale bar = 5 µm.)

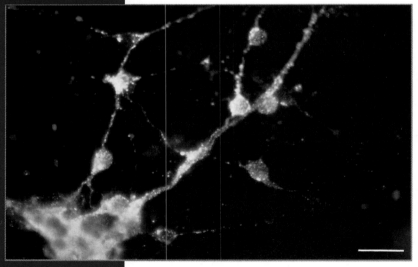

Figure 6—Rabies virus–infected rat cultured neurons from cerebral cortex. Day 6 postinfection. Viral inclusions are visualized with a fluorescein-isothiocyanate–labeled anti–rabies virus nucleocapsid polyclonal serum. (Scale bar = 10 µm.)

dysfunction.[10,30] During experimental rabies infection of the mouse (with a fixed strain), it was shown that the electroencephalographic recording is altered very early, even before the first clinical signs occur.[31] These alterations include changes in the regulation of sleep stages, the disappearance of paradoxical sleep, and pseudoperiodic facial myoclonus. Such alterations are followed by an electroencephalographic slowing, accompanied by a flattening of cortical activity. In the agonal phase, the brain's electric activity stops about 30 minutes before cardiac arrest, suggesting that cardiac failure is not the direct origin of rabies death. When electroencephalographic recordings and analysis were performed on mice infected with a street strain of virus,[32] different patterns of evolution were observed, suggesting that different pathogenetic mechanisms occur for different strains. However, these data support the idea that rabies may be a disease of impaired information transmission.

In past years, several studies have concentrated on events that could affect neurotransmitter metabolism, release, binding, and uptake during rabies infection. In vitro, impairments in the binding of an antagonist to muscarinic acetylcholine receptor[33] and impairments in gamma-aminobutyric acid (GABA) release and uptake by primary neuronal cultures[34] have been shown. In vivo, alterations have been described in neurotransmitter receptors (e.g., 5-hydroxytryptamine [5-HT] receptors[35]) as well as in neurotransmitter release (5-HT[36]). Taken together, these studies demonstrate that the rabies-induced neural dysfunctions do not proceed through a common mechanism (e.g., general breakdown of neuronal syntheses) but through a selective one. Until now, the alterations that have been reported may have explained some of the rabies-induced clinical manifestations (anxiety and aggressiveness) but not the rabies death.

IMMUNOPATHOLOGY

Although not discussed in detail in this

chapter, rabies-induced immunopathology must be considered. Important hallmarks of rabies pathogenesis include the role of the rabies nucleocapsid as a superantigen in humans and mice,[37] the rabies-induced immunosuppression, the "early death" phenomenon, and the peripheral immunopathogenesis that is responsible for hindlimb paralysis.[38] However, it is still difficult to determine a mechanism for correlating these events with the neural dysfunctions and clinical signs.[39] In this regard, recent reports that mention alterations in cytokine (IL-1, TNF-α) syntheses and binding to cytokine receptors[40,41] during experimentally induced rabies in rodents offer new perspectives on rabies-induced impairments affecting the immune and nervous systems.

PATHOGENESIS OF RABIES-RELATED VIRUSES

Among the *Lyssavirus* genus of the Rhabdoviridae family, rabies has been classified as genotype 1, whereas the rabies-related viruses, that is, Lagos bat lyssavirus, Mokola bat lyssavirus, Duvenhage bat lyssavirus, European bat lyssavirus 1 (EBL1), European bat lyssavirus 2 (EBL2), and the recently reported Australian bat lyssavirus (ABLV),[42] have been classified respectively in genotypes 2 to 7. A few pathogenetic studies concern the latter three lyssaviruses. It has been hypothesized that Mokola, Lagos, and Duvenhage rabies-related viruses could behave as rabies virus for viral spread via neural pathways, with replication in neurons and peripheral dissemination to organs outside of the CNS, but with some variations and with more pronounced CNS lesions (perivascular cuffing, neuronal degeneration).[4]

CLINICAL DISEASE IN HUMANS AND ANIMALS

The clinical symptoms of rabies in humans (discussed in Drs. McQuiston and Child's paper on p. 27) are similar in many respects to the signs observed in animals (discussed in Dr. Chomel's paper on p. 20).

In fact, it should be considered that the clinical features of human rabies represent just one example among mammals. For instance, two thirds of human rabies patients suffer from the furious form of rabies and the remaining one third suffer from the paralytic form[39]; in dogs, however, the dumb form of rabies is more common (even if the aggressive stage is frequent and very pronounced), and the furious form is almost always seen in cats. Clinical manifestations among different animals vary widely, depending on a variety of factors, including the viral strain, the animal host, the virus localization, and the host immune response.[39] A distinctive feature of human rabies may be hydrophobia, which is not seen in dogs; during the disease dogs try to drink water, but they are unable to swallow because of the paralysis.

CENTRIFUGAL SPREAD TO PERIPHERAL TISSUES

While viral dissemination occurs in the CNS, infection of neurons from the motor neurons of the brain stem and spinal cord is followed by replication of virus in these neurons and a subsequent anterograde axonal transport in peripheral nerves to a variety of tissues. As seen in the centripetal and intra-CNS spread of the rabies virus, this transport can be prevented by colchicine, meaning that it is microtubule-dependent.[17] This viral dissemination allows infection of peripheral tissues such as muscle fibers, salivary glands, corneas, adrenal medullae, lacrimal glands, myocardium, kidneys, lungs, pancreas, and epidermis.[4,24] Infection of salivary glands is of special importance because it allows further transmission of the disease for many species.

RABIES RESERVOIRS: THE CARRIER STATE

A major concern in rabies transmission in wildlife is the search for reservoir species. In the past, it has been hypothesized that small rodents or even arthropods could play

Hallmarks of rabies pathogenesis include the role of the rabies nucleocapsid as a superantigen, the rabies-induced immunosuppression, the "early death" phenomenon, the neuronal dysfunction, and the peripheral immunopathogenesis responsible for hindlimb paralysis.

such a role, but no evidence to support this theory has ever been found. In North America, bats have been thought to be a reservoir species[43] because they fulfill most of the required criteria: They are able to harbor a wide variety of viral strains, they are widely distributed, and they are able to migrate over long distances. The other main reservoir species are the raccoon, skunk, red fox, and arctic fox.[44] In other parts of the world, main rabies vectors such as the fox (Europe) or the dog (Asia or Africa) would be able, by incubating the disease for long periods, to generate new rabies foci, even in places where rabies was thought to be under control.[45] This would allow virus survival for long periods between epizootic outbreaks. Another way for an animal species to act as a reservoir would be to become immune after infection while continuing to shed virus. This "carrier state" refers to an animal with a chronic infection, with or without a period of clinical signs, even though it can still transmit the disease generally by excretion of virus in saliva. To test this hypothesis, Fekadu and coworkers experimentally infected dogs with two street rabies strains[46,47]; viral shedding was observed in the saliva of some of the dogs for up to 14 days before clinical signs appeared. In this experiment, some dogs recovered, and one of them intermittently excreted rabies virus in its saliva for up to 305 days after complete recovery. Because at necropsy viable virus was found in the palatine tonsils of this dog[48] and in those of street rabies–infected laboratory animals (dogs, monkeys, foxes), the palatine tonsils rather than the submaxillary salivary glands have been thought to act as a possible sequestration site. Such a long time between the beginning and end of viral shedding is uncommon and would be linked to the characteristics of specific street rabies strains: The 10-day observation period observed by the United States and most other countries is sufficient, as these cases are unusual. These experimental data may be connected to the carrier states that have been reported in dogs in Ethiopia[49] or India[50]; however, additional experiments with modern techniques are still required to test this hypothesis. Until now, no convincing data have been reported regarding the carrier state in naturally occurring rabies in North America.[24]

SUMMARY

Among neurotropic viruses, rabies virus shows the distinctive feature of using axonal transport almost exclusively for dissemination and for induction of major neural dysfunctions without gross neuronal lesions. Knowledge of the different mechanisms of CNS rabies pathogenesis (spread, tropism, neural dysfunction) provides perspectives in using pharmacologic means in addition to the classic vaccinotherapy to combat these events in rabies (and rabies-related) virus infections.

ACKNOWLEDGMENTS

The author thanks H. Tsiang for helpful comments and M.H. Matuszewski and R. Etessami for help in preparing the manuscript. Part of this work was supported by grants from the D.R.E.T. (contract no. 95/178) and C.N.R.S. (contract no. 96/C/07).

REFERENCES

1. Matsumoto S: Electron microscopy of nerve cells infected with street rabies virus. *Virology* 17:198–202, 1962.
2. Tordo N, Poch O: Structure of rabies virus, in Campbell JB, Charlton KM (eds): *Rabies.* Boston, Kluwer Academic Publ, 1988, pp 25–45.
3. Baer GM: *The Natural History of Rabies,* ed 2. CRC Press, Boca Raton, 1991.
4. Charlton KM: The pathogenesis of rabies and other lyssaviral infections: Recent studies. In Rupprecht CE, Dietzschold B, Koprowski H (eds): *Lyssaviruses.* Berlin, Springer-Verlag, 1994, pp 95–115.
5. Shankar V, Dietzschold B, Koprowski H: Direct entry of rabies virus into the central nervous system without prior local replication. *J Virol* 65(5): 2736–2738, 1991.
6. Murphy FA, Bauer SP, Harrison AK, Winn WC Jr: Comparative pathogenesis of rabies and rabies-like viruses. Viral infection and transit from inoculation site to the central nervous system. *Lab Invest* 28:361, 1973.
7. Charlton KM, Casey GA: Experimental rabies in skunks: Immunofluorescent, light and electron microscopic studies. *Lab Invest* 41:36–44, 1979.
8. Tsiang H, Koenig J: Different behaviour of fixed and street rabies virus strains in cultured rat myo-

tubes, in Mahy B, Kolakofsky D (eds): *The Biology of Negative Strand Viruses.* Amsterdam, Elsevier, 1987, pp 363–368.

9. Tsiang H, DeLaporte S, Ambroise DJ, et al: Infection of cultured rat myotubes and neurons from the spinal cord by rabies virus. *J Neuropathol Exp Neurol* 5:28–42, 1986.

10. Tsiang H: Interactions of rabies virus and host cells, in Campbell JB, Charlton KM (eds): *Rabies.* Boston, Kluwer Academic Publ, 1988, pp 67–100.

11. Lentz TH, Burrage TG, Smith AL, et al: Is the acetylcholine receptor a rabies virus receptor? *Science* 215:182–184, 1982.

12. Thoulouze MI, Lafage M, Schachner M, et al: The neural cell adhesion molecule is a receptor for rabies virus. *J Virol* 72(9):7181–7190, 1998.

13. Tsiang H, Derer M, Taxi J: An in vivo and in vitro study of rabies virus infection of the rat superior cervical ganglia. *Arch Virol* 76:231–243, 1983.

14. Gaudin Y, Ruigrok RWH, Knossow M, Flamand A: Low-pH conformational changes of rabies virus glycoprotein and their role in membrane fusion *J Virol* 67:1365–1372, 1993.

15. Coulon P, Derbin C, Kucera P, et al: Invasion of the peripheral nervous systems of adult mice by the CVS strain of rabies virus and its avirulent derivative Av01. *J Virol* 63:3550–3554, 1989.

16. Bijlenga G, Heany T: Post-exposure local treatment of mice infected with rabies with two axonal flow inhibitors, colchicine and vinblastine. *J Gen Virol* 39:381–385, 1978.

17. Tsiang H: Evidence for intraaxonal transport of fixed and street rabies virus. *J Neuropathol Exp Neurol* 38:286–296, 1979.

18. Tsiang H, Ceccaldi PE, Lycke E: Rabies virus infection and transport in human sensory dorsal root ganglia neurons. *J Gen Virol* 72:1191–1194, 1991.

19. Lycke E, Tsiang H: Rabies virus infection of cultured rat sensory neurons. *J Virol* 61(9):2733–2741, 1987.

20. Tsiang H, Lycke E, Ceccaldi PE, et al: The anterograde transport of rabies virus in rat sensory dorsal roo ganglia neurons. *J Gen Virol* 70:2075–2085, 1989.

21. Kucera P, Dolivo M, Coulon P, Flamand A: Pathways of the early propagation of virulent and avirulent rabies virus strains from the eye to the brain. *J Virol* 55:158–162, 1985.

22. Gillet JP, Derer P, Tsiang H: Axonal transport of rabies virus in the central nervous system of the rat. *J Neuropathol Exp Neurol* 45(6):619–634, 1986.

23. Ceccaldi PE, Gillet JP, Tsiang H: Inhibition of the transport of rabies virus in the central nervous system. *J Neuropathol Exp Neurol* 48(6):620–630, 1989.

24. Charlton KM: The pathogenesis of rabies, in Campbell JB, Charlton KM (eds): *Rabies.* Boston, Kluwer Academic Publ, 1988, pp 101–150.

25. Schneider LG: Spread of virus from the CNS, in Baer GM (ed): *The Natural History of Rabies,* vol 1. New York, Academic Publ, 1975, pp 199–216.

26. Graham D, Lantis PL: *Greenfield's Neuropathology,* ed 6, vol 2. London, Arnold, 1981.

27. Tsiang H, Koulakoff A, Bizzini B, Berwald-Netter Y: Neurotropism of rabies virus, an in vitro study. *J Neuropathol Exp Neurol* 42(4):439–452, 1983.

28. Jackson AC, Park M: Apoptotic cell death in experimental rabies in suckling mice. *Acta Neuropathol* 95:159–164, 1998.

29. Charlton KM, Casey GA, Webster WA, Bundza A: Experimental rabies in skunks and foxes, pathogenesis of the spongiform lesions. *Lab Invest* 57(6):634–645, 1987.

30. Tsiang H: Pathophysiology of rabies virus infection of the nervous system. *Adv Virus Res* 42:375–412, 1993.

31. Gourmelon P, Briet D, Court L, Tsiang H: Electrophysiological and sleep alterations in experimental mouse rabies. *Brain Res* 398:128–140, 1986.

32. Gourmelon P, Briet D, Clarendon D, et al: Sleep alterations in experimental street rabies virus infection occur in the absence of major EEG abnormalities. *Brain Res* 554:159–165, 1991.

33. Tsiang H: An in vitro study of rabies pathogenesis. *Bull Inst Past* 83:41–56, 1985.

34. Ladogana A, Bouzamondo E, Pocchiari M, Tsiang H: Modification of tritiated (-amino-*n*-butyric acid transport in rabies virus–infected primary cortical cultures. *J Gen Virol* 75:623.

35. Ceccaldi PE, Fillion MP, Ermine A, et al: Rabies virus selectively alters 5-HT receptor subtypes in rat brain. *Eur J Pharmacol-Molec Pharmacol Section* 245:129–138, 1993.

36. Bouzamondo E, Ladogana A, Tsiang H: Alteration of potassium-evoked 5-HT release from virus-infected rat cortical synaptosomes. *Neuroreport* 4:555–558, 1993.

37. Lafon M, Lafage M, Martinez-Arends A, et al: Evidence for a viral superantigen in humans. *Nature* 358:507–509, 1992.

38. Weiland F, Cox JH, Meyer S, et al: Rabies virus neuritic paralysis: Immunopathogenesis of nonfatal paralytic rabies. *J Virol* 66(8):5096–5099, 1992.

39. Hemachudha T: Human rabies: Clinical aspects, pathogenesis and potential therapy, in Rupprecht CE, Dietzschold B, Koprowski H (eds): *Lyssaviruses.* Berlin, Springer Verlag, 1994, pp 121–140.

40. Marquette C, Ceccaldi PE, Ban E, et al: Alteration of interleukin-1α production and interleukin-1α binding sites in mouse brain during rabies infection. *Arch Virol* 141:573–585, 1996.

41. Marquette C, Van Dam AM, Ceccaldi PE, et al: Induction of immunoreactive interleukin-1β and tumor necrosis factor-α in the brains of rabies virus infected rats. *J Neuroimmunol* 68:45–51, 1996.

42. Gould AR, Hyatt AD, Lunt R, et al: Characterisation of a novel lyssavirus isolated from *Pteropid* bats in Australia. *Virus Res* 54:165–187, 1998.

43. Tinline RR: Persistence of rabies in wildlife, in: Campbell JB, Charlton KM (eds): *Rabies.* Boston, Kluwer Academic Publ, 1988, pp 301–322.

44. Krebs JW, Smith JS, Rupprecht CE, Childs IE: Rabies surveillance in the United States during 1996. *JAVMA* 211(12):1525–1539, 1997.

45. Blancou I: Epizootiology of rabies: Eurasia and Africa, in: Campbell JB, Charlton KM (eds): *Rabies.* Boston, Kluwer Academic Publ, 1988, pp 243–265.

46. Fekadu M, Shaddock JH, Baer GM: Excretion of rabies virus in the saliva of dogs. *J Infect Dis* 145:715, 1982.

47. Fekadu M, Shaddock JH, Baer GM: Intermittent excretion of rabies virus in the saliva of a dog two and six months after it had recovered from experimental rabies. *Am J Trop Med Hyg* 30:1113, 1981.

48. Fekadu M, Shaddock JH, Chandler FW, Baer GM: Rabies virus in the tonsils of a carrier dog. *Arch Virol* 78:37, 1983.

49. Fekadu M: Atypical rabies in dogs in Ethiopia. *Ethiop Med J* 10:79–86, 1972.

50. Veeraraghavan N: Studies in the salivary excretion of rabies virus by the dog from Surrandi. Paris, Pasteur Institute, Annual Report of the Director, 1968.

Rabies Exposure and Clinical Disease in Animals

Bruno B. Chomel, DVM, PhD

Associate Professor of Zoonoses, Department of Population Health and Reproduction
Director, Masters of Preventive Veterinary Medicine Program
Director, WHO/PAHO Collaborating Center on Emerging Zoonoses, School of Veterinary Medicine
University of California, Davis, California

R ABIES MAY HAVE EXISTED IN NORTH AMERICA BEFORE THE EUROPEAN COLONIZA-TION AND THE IMPORTATION OF DOMESTIC ANIMALS INCUBATING THE DISEASE. IF VAMPIRE BAT RABIES WAS ALREADY ASSOCIATED WITH HUMAN ILLNESS AT THE TIME OF THE SPANISH CONQUEST, THE FIRST INDICATION OF RABIES IN TERRESTRIAL MAMMALS WAS RE-PORTED IN WHAT IS NOW CALIFORNIA.[1] UNTIL THE MIDDLE OF THE 20TH CENTURY, RABIES IN NORTH AMERICA WAS MAINLY ASSOCIATED WITH ITS CANINE RESERVOIR, DESPITE OUTBREAKS RE-PORTED IN FOXES IN THE MID-ATLANTIC COLONIES DURING THE 18TH CENTURY AND REPORTS OF SKUNK RABIES IN THE WESTERN STATES BY THE 19TH CENTURY.[1] RABIES BECAME A NATIONAL-LY REPORTABLE DISEASE IN THE UNITED STATES IN 1938, AND BY 1960 RABIES WAS DIAGNOSED MORE FREQUENTLY AMONG WILDLIFE THAN AMONG DOMESTICATED ANIMALS (FIGURE 1).[2] BY 1981 THE ANNUAL NUMBER OF RABIES CASES REPORTED IN DOMESTIC CATS IN THE UNITED STATES EXCEEDED THOSE REPORTED IN DOMESTIC DOGS (TABLE 1).

RABIES IN DOMESTIC ANIMALS
Dogs

The dog is certainly a major species associated with rabies and its transmission to humans. Fortunately, rabies is now a rare disease in humans in the United States. Since canine rabies has been controlled, the incidence of human rabies, excluding cases acquired abroad and cases trans-mitted by bats, has fallen from 43 (0.03 per 100,000) in 1945 to less than 1 per year (<0.001 per 100,000) in the 1980s and 1990s. Rabies in the United States is mainly a wildlife disease affect-ing raccoons, skunks, coyotes, foxes, and bats (Table 1). However, humans are still probably at greater risk of acquiring rabies from a rabid dog, as dogs account for a large majority of bite in-cidents reported in this country. In a review of dog rabies cases in 1988 in the United States,[3] most canine rabies cases occurred in young dogs (57% in dogs ≤1 year), dogs considered as pets (84% of the cases), and mostly those from a rural environment (85%). More importantly, virtu-ally all rabid dogs were never vaccinated or their vaccination status was unknown.

There was an average of 148 rabid dogs (range of 111 to 182) per year for the 10-year peri-od of 1987 through 1996 (Table 1). In 1996, Texas reported the largest number of cases of ra-bies in dogs (15 cases), 6 of which were associated with the ongoing epizootic of rabies in dogs

Humans are probably at greater risk of acquiring rabies from a rabid dog.

and coyotes in southern Texas. Other than Texas, Georgia (8 cases), Iowa (12 cases), North Carolina (10 cases), South Dakota (8 cases), Tennessee (6 cases), and Puerto Rico (12 cases) were the only states/territories with more than 5 cases.[4]

When introduced to a victim by a bite, the rabies virus will multiply locally at the wound site and then will invade the peripheral nerve(s) supplying that area.[5] The virus migrates along the nerves to reach the central nervous system and radiates further through the nerves in various organs, including the salivary glands. The virus is shed in the saliva and can be transmitted to a new victim through a bite. The incubation of rabies varies from a few days to several months, and the virus can be shed in the saliva a few days prior to the appearance of any clinical neurologic signs. This is the main reason why a dog that bites a human is quarantined for 10 days. If the dog is healthy 10 days after the bite incident, one can assume that the dog was not shedding the virus at the time of the bite, and, consequently, the bite victim does not need a rabies postexposure treatment (a series of five doses of 1.0 ml of vaccine by the intramuscular route on days 0, 3, 7, 14, and 28).

Rabies is characterized mainly by neurologic and behavioral disorders. During the initial prodromic phase the dog is anxious and nervous and suffers from changes in personality. After 2 or 3 days the furious or

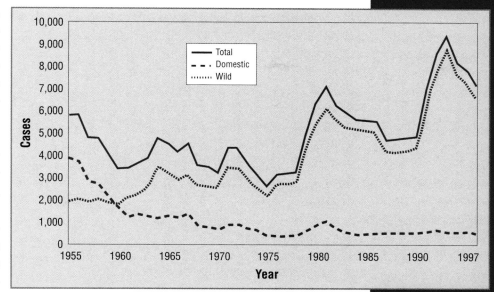

Figure 1—Cases of animal rabies in the United States by year, 1955 to 1997.[4]

TABLE 1
Reported Rabies Cases in the United States by Type of Animal, 1980–1996

| Year | Domestic Animals | | | | Wildlife | | | | |
	Dogs	Cats	Horses	Ruminants	Raccoons	Skunks	Foxes	Coyotes	Bats
1980	247	214	NA	NA	394	4,096	213	NA	726
1981	216	285	NA	NA	481	4,480	196	NA	858
1982	153	209	NA	NA	1,156	3,088	222	NA	975
1983	132	169	64	217	1,906	2,285	111	1	909
1984	97	140	55	159	1,820	2,082	139	2	1,038
1985	113	130	38	220	1,487	2,507	181	2	830
1986	95	166	43	210	1,576	2,379	207	6	788
1987	170	166	39	182	1,311	2,033	119	1	629
1988	128	192	43	180	1,463	1,791	183	7	638
1989	160	212	51	159	1,544	1,657	207	7	720
1990	148	176	45	182	1,821	1,579	197	7	637
1991	155	189	44	227	3,079	2,073	318	50	690
1992	182	290	49	207	4,311	2,334	397	75	647
1993	130	291	48	135	5,912	1,640	361	74	759
1994	153	267	42	126	4,780	1,450	535	85	631
1995	146	288	43	148	3,964	1,774	513	83	787
1996	111	266	46	147	3,395	1,656	412	23	741

NA = not available.
Source: Centers for Disease Control and Prevention, Viral and Rickettsial Zoonoses Branch data.

paralytic form starts. In the furious form, which lasts 1 to 7 days, the dog shows irritability, aggression, hypersensitivity, disorientation, and sometimes grand mal seizures. In the paralytic or dumb form, which lasts 1 to 10 days, paralysis will affect one or more limbs. Paralysis then progresses to affect the entire nervous system. Cranial nerve paralysis, especially laryngeal paralysis, is often the first recognized sign. Death occurs within 10 days.

Prevention of dog rabies is based on vaccination of susceptible animals, confinement of animals, quarantine of dogs that bite, and removal of stray animals. Recommendations for state and local rabies vaccination and control measures are published yearly by the National Association of State Public Health Veterinarians. All states require rabies vaccination in dogs. Interstate travel usually requires possession of a health certificate and a proof of rabies vaccination. Seventeen rabies vaccines are currently marketed for dogs in the United States and should be administered according to the manufacturer's instructions. Puppies should be vaccinated at 3 months of age and revaccinated 1 year later at 15 months, after which they should receive annual or triennial boosters. If dogs with a current rabies immunization are exposed to a rabid animal, they should be revaccinated immediately and then confined and observed for 90 days. Unvaccinated animals are usually euthanized or may be placed in strict isolation for 6 months and vaccinated 1 month before release.[5]

Cats

In the United States, feline rabies cases have surpassed those in dogs, sometimes by twofold, every year since 1981. For the 10-year period of 1987 to 1996, a yearly average of 234 rabid cats (range of 166 to 291) was reported (Table 1). Most of these feline cases occurred in geographic areas experiencing epizootics of rabies in raccoons, with remaining cases associated with those of ra-

bid skunks in the Central Plain states.[4] Rabies is difficult to diagnose in cats in the early stages. Major signs of rabies in cats reported by veterinarians include behavior change, gait abnormality, strange or unusual look in the eyes, and a reported wound within the preceding 6 months.[6] Owners also often report increased frequency of vocalization. In a study of 10 rabid cats from Maryland, incubation periods ranged from 2 to 12 weeks, with a median of 4 to 6 weeks.[6] Several mid-Atlantic states have passed laws to make cat rabies vaccination mandatory. Several vaccines are licensed in the United States for cat immunization, and one newly approved vaccine can be used at 8 weeks of age.

Ferrets

Like other carnivores, ferrets are susceptible to rabies. Experimentally induced rabies with a skunk strain in ferrets was characterized by an incubation period of 33 days (range of 16 to 96 days).[7] Clinical signs included ascending paralysis, ataxia, cachexia, bladder atony, fever, hyperactivity, tremors, and paresthesia. Most of the ferrets died in 4 to 5 days (range of 2 to 10 days) after the onset of clinical signs.[7] In the United States, only 23 cases of rabies in domestic ferrets have been reported since 1958, most often in pet ferrets, some of which were acquired from pet shops.[7,8] Rabies immunization of ferrets with an inactivated vaccine (Imrab® 3 [Merial]) has been shown to be effective for at least a year.[8] On February 8, 1990, the U.S. Department of Agriculture granted approval for the use of this vaccine in ferrets at 3 months of age or more. Annual booster vaccinations are required. Since 1998 the National Association of State Public Health Veterinarians in its *Compendium of Animal Rabies Control* recommends that postexposure management in ferrets be the same as in dogs and cats. Therefore the previous requirement that all ferrets that have bitten humans be killed and their brains examined for rabies is no longer applicable.[9]

Horses

Although the incidence of rabies in horses is low (<1% of all diagnosed rabid animals), approximately 45 to 50 cases of equine rabies are reported annually in the United States (Table 1).[10] Over 700 cases were reported in southern Ontario between 1970 and 1990. Rabies cases in horses are usually caused by strains associated with the main terrestrial reservoirs of rabies in North America. For instance, in the northeastern United States and southern Canada, cases are associated with skunk and fox strains, whereas in the southeastern and Atlantic regions of the United States they involve raccoon strains. In the central United States and California, skunks are the main rabies reservoir. Bat rabies, widespread throughout North America, can also be transmitted accidentally to horses.

A spectrum of clinical signs, ranging from paralysis to abnormal behavior, has been reported in rabid horses. Neurologic disorders in horses may involve several other infectious diseases other than rabies, such as equine encephalitides. Exposure of horses to a suspected rabid animal is also rarely witnessed. Because of the lack of pathognomonic signs, rabies is often suspected late in the clinical evolution of the disease and the number of persons exposed to a rabid horse is often high; postexposure treatment of several dozen persons is quite common. Fortunately, no human death from contamination by a rabid horse has occurred in North America. In horses rabies incubation averages 2 to 4 weeks (range of 2 weeks to 3 months). Clinical signs of disease at the time of initial examination usually include weakness of the hindquarters (ataxia and paresis), lameness, and colic.[11] After an excitation period, paralytic signs occur that cause difficulty in swallowing, followed by incoordination of the extremities. In all cases there is a change in behavior. Because neurologic signs always progress with rabies, other possibilities should be considered if clinical signs have not worsened in 5 days. Usually,

horses die within a week. It is generally recommended that horses be vaccinated against rabies in endemic areas. Because many horses are kept as pets or are in close contact with humans, vaccination of horses may serve to establish an immune barrier between humans and the wildlife population by decreasing the frequency of rabies in horses. Five inactivated rabies vaccines (in combination or not) are licensed in the United States for use in horses.[9] Horses must be 3 months or older at primary vaccination and must receive a booster dose annually.

Cattle and Small Ruminants

Since 1990, the number of rabid ruminants in the United States has exceeded the number of rabid dogs every year, with the exception of 1994 (Table 1). Cattle account for the majority of these cases. Distribution of rabies cases in cattle followed that of skunks in the central United States and raccoons in the northeast/mid-Atlantic region. In 1996, Iowa (37 cases), South Dakota (16 cases), and Texas (10 cases) reported the largest numbers of rabid cattle.[4] On average, fewer than a dozen sheep and even fewer goats are reported rabid every year. A few cases have been reported in llamas in the United States. Rabies in cattle is characterized by a long incubation period, 14 to 26 days in 14 cows infected experimentally with a European red fox strain[12] and 15 days in 18 cows infected experimentally with a North American rabies strain.[13] The first observed signs in these experimentally infected cows were hypersalivation and loss of appetite, as well as behavioral change. Muzzle tremors were observed in 80% of the animals. After a few days, anorexia, foamy hypersalivation, and loss of weight were reported. Voice modification (bellowing), digestive signs such as such as tenesmus and constipation, and paresis or paralysis occurred 2 days after initial signs. In cows inoculated with the North American strain, 70% showed aggressiveness, hyperexcitability, and/or hyperesthesia, whereas none of the cows inoculated with the Euro-

It is generally recommended that horses be vaccinated against rabies in endemic areas.

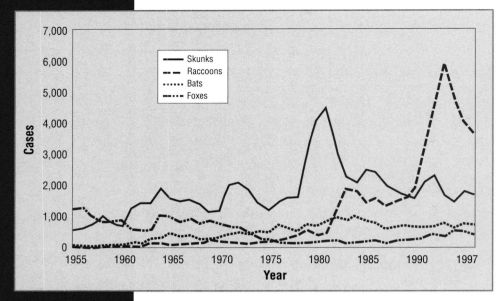

Figure 2—Cases of rabies in wild animals in the United States, by year and species, 1955 to 1997.[4]

pean strain showed signs of aggression. The cows died within a week (mean 4–5 days, range 1–8 days). Presence of the three major symptoms, hypersalivation, loss of appetite, and frequent mooing, should always suggest rabies infection. Rabies vaccination of cattle in rabies-endemic areas may be warranted.

RABIES IN WILDLIFE
Raccoons

Since 1990 raccoons *(Procyon lotor)* account for the largest proportion of rabies cases in one animal species (Figure 2). In 1996 raccoons were the most frequently reported rabid wildlife species (50.4% of all animal cases and 55% of all wildlife cases). Most (99.1% in 1996) of the rabid raccoons are reported in the mid-Atlantic and northeastern states (18 states and the District of Columbia in 1996), where the raccoon rabies epizootic has been spreading since it was introduced in the late 1970s by the translocation of infected animals to stock hunting clubs from a southeastern focus of the disease (Figure 3).[2] No clear seasonal, sexual, or age-related factors have been definitively identified. The distribution of rabies in raccoons in the United States shows that urban and suburban areas continue to be intensely affected.[14] Raccoons, unlike other well-known rabies reservoirs such as skunks and foxes, have adapted successfully to urban/

suburban environments, typically achieving their greatest densities where humans reside. It is difficult to determine the duration of the incubation period in wildlife, but it is estimated that the average incubation period is 3 to 4 weeks (range of 10 to 107 days). Rabid raccoons may exhibit aggressive behavior in 30% to 50% of the cases and can be observed roaming in yards during daylight in 25% to 40% of the cases.[15] In about 10% of the cases the raccoons reportedly appear to be sick, with incoordination or paralysis. Contamination of domestic animals occurs after a rabid raccoon has bitten a domestic animal, more likely a ruminant or a horse, or when a stray or free-roaming cat or sometimes a dog has been involved in a fight with a rabid raccoon. The high density of the raccoon population in suburban areas explains the high number of rabies cases and the frequent exposure of domestic cats to rabid animals. Oral vaccination of raccoons is now underway in Massachusetts, New York, New Jersey, Florida, Vermont, Maryland, and Ohio to reduce the spread of the disease.[4]

Skunks

Skunk rabies has been reported in parts of North America since the late 1800s and early 1900s in the midwestern and western United States. It is mainly found in three different regions: North Central from Alberta (Canada) to Tennessee, West in California, and South Central from Nebraska and Missouri to Texas (Figure 3).[14] In southern Ontario, Quebec, and upper New York state, rabid skunks are infected with the fox rabies variant.[14] In infected areas, a 6- to 8-year epidemic cycle has been recorded. Most of the cases are reported in early spring and late summer, related to breeding season in February and March and dispersal of the young animals in the fall. Skunk rabies mainly affects the striped skunk *(Mephitis mephitis)*. Skunks accounted for

23.2% of rabid animals reported in 1996.[4] Clinical signs of rabies in skunks are very similar to what has been presented for raccoons. In experimentally infected animals restlessness in the early stage of the disease is very common. Paralysis develops in a few days, and the animals die usually within a week. Of domestic animal rabies cases, cattle cases are most commonly associated with skunk rabies. Distribution of rabies cases in cattle closely follows that of skunks in the central United States, raccoons in the northeast/mid-Atlantic region, and coyotes, foxes, and skunks in Texas.

Foxes

Foxes represent the main rabies reservoir in eastern Canada and Alaska. A spillover of the eastern Canada red fox *(Vulpes vulpes)* epidemic has been intermittently affecting the New England states (Figure 3).[4] In Alaska and the Canadian Arctic (Northwest Territories), polar foxes *(Alopex lagopus)* are infected with a polar fox strain of rabies virus. Two rabies virus variants have been identified in persistent foci in gray foxes *(Urocyon cinereoargenteus)* in Arizona and Texas.[4] In the United States foxes accounted for almost 6% of the rabies cases in animals reported in 1996, with most of the fox cases occurring in the eastern coastal states and being caused probably by spillover from infected raccoons.[4] Successful oral vaccination programs have been conducted in red foxes in eastern Canada, especially Ontario, and such programs are considered for control of Arctic fox rabies.

Coyotes

Prior to 1988 rabies was reported only sporadically in coyotes, usually as a spillover of the epizootic in skunks or raccoons. In late 1988 an epizootic of canine rabies in which coyotes *(Canis latrans)* were the primary vector but that involved coyotes and domestic dogs started in southern Texas along the Mexican border (Figure 3). It expanded at a rate of 70 to 80 km per year during the following years to reach 18 counties by 1994. More than 500 rabies cases (270 coyotes, 216 dogs) were related to that epidemic between 1988 and 1994.[16] In 1996, 19 of the 25 coyote cases reported to the Centers for Disease Control and Prevention (CDC) were from southern Texas.[4] Because of that epidemic, more than 2,000 people in southern Texas received postexposure rabies treatment and 2 persons died of rabies. An oral rabies vaccination program using a rabies vaccinia recombinant vaccine was implemented in 1995, and several million doses have been distributed in southern Texas since then.

Bats

Bat rabies in nonhematophagous bats is widespread in North America. Since the transmission of rabies by a bat was first reported in 1953, when a young boy was bitten by a rabid bat in Tampa, Florida, an average of 700 to 800 rabid insectivorous bats have been reported yearly in the United States from all of the 48 contiguous states. Bat rabies accounted for 10.4% of all cases of rabies in animals reported in 1996, with California and Texas accounting for a third of the 741 cases reported that year.[4] Rabies has been diagnosed in a wide range of insectivorous bat species (virtually all species of North

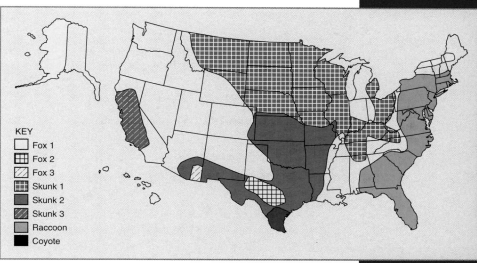

Figure 3—
Distribution of
major terrestrial
reservoirs of rabies
in the United
States.[4]

American bats), but most of the epidemiologic data available concern colonial bats, Mexican free-tail bats *(Tadarida brasiliensis mexicana),* and the big brown bat *(Eptesicus fuscus).* The incidence of rabies is slightly higher in colonial species (59%) than in solitary species (41%).[17] After an incubation of 3 to 12 weeks, experimentally infected bats infrequently develop an aggressive behavior. Rabid bats are more likely to be found on the ground, unable to fly, with an apparent paralysis. Domestic animals can accidentally become infected with bat rabies virus strains. Cats are particularly at risk of exposure when playing with a sick bat that they may have found on the ground or on the floor inside a house. It is therefore highly recommended that cats, even if kept strictly indoors, be vaccinated against rabies in areas where bat rabies is endemic. It is also important to emphasize the risk for humans exposed to rabid bats. Between 1980 and 1990, 32 humans died of rabies in the United States, of whom 20 acquired their infection in the country. Seventeen of these 20 autochthonous cases were identified by genetic analysis to be variants associated with rabies in bats.[4]

Mongooses

Rabies cases are regularly diagnosed in mongooses *(Herpestes auropunctatus)* in Puerto Rico. The small Indian mongoose was introduced in many of the Caribbean Islands for rodent control in the sugar cane fields during the last third of the 19th century. Mongooses are now an important rabies reservoir in Cuba, the Dominican Republic, Haiti, Grenada, and Puerto Rico.[18] Between 25 and 50 rabies cases in mongooses in Puerto Rico are reported annually to the CDC. Molecular epidemiology methods (sequence analysis) have shown that the mongoose rabies isolates originated from dog rabies strains, which have been endemic in the Caribbean for centuries.[19] Rabid mongooses are easily identified, as they are very aggressive and are often seen attacking domestic animals. When caged, they will furiously attack

the wire mesh, emitting a prolonged high-pitched shriek and frequently damaging their snout and teeth in attempts to bite the cage.[18]

REFERENCES

1. Baer GM: Rabies—An historical perspective. *Infect Agents Dis* 3:168–180, 1994.
2. Rupprecht CE, Smith JS, Fekadu M, Childs JE: The ascension of wildlife rabies: A cause for public health concern or intervention? *Emerg Infect Dis* 1(4):107–114, 1995.
3. Eng TR, Fishbein DB: National Study Group on Rabies: Epidemiologic factors, clinical findings, and vaccination status of rabies in cats and dogs in the United States in 1988. *JAVMA* 197:201–209, 1990.
4. Krebs JW, Smith JS, Rupprecht CE, Childs JE: Rabies surveillance in the United States during 1997. *JAVMA* 213(12):1714–1715, 1998.
5. Chomel BB: Appendix A: Zoonotic diseases: From dogs to people, in Siegal MS (ed): *U.C. Davis Book of Dogs: A Complete Medical Reference Guide for Dogs and Puppies.* New York, Harper Collins Publishers, 1995, pp 469–476.
6. Fogelman V, Fischman HR, Horman JT, Girgor JK: Epidemiologic and clinical characteristics of rabies in cats. *JAVMA* 202(11):1829–1833, 1993.
7. Niezgoda M, Briggs DJ, Shaddock J, et al: Pathogenesis of experimentally induced rabies in domestic ferrets. *Am J Vet Res* 58:1327–1331, 1997.
8. Rupprecht CE, Gilbert J, Pitts R, et al: Evaluation of an inactivated rabies virus vaccine in domestic ferrets. *JAVMA* 196:1614–1616, 1990.
9. National Association of State Public Health Veterinarians: 1998. Compendium of animal rabies control. *MMWR* 47:RR-9:1–9, 1998.
10. Chomel BB: Appendix A: Zoonotic diseases: From horses to people, in Siegal MS (ed): *U.C. Davis Book of Horses, A Complete Medical Reference Guide for Horses and Foals.* New York, Harper Collins Publishers, 1996, pp 411–416.
11. Green SL, Smith LL, Vernau W, Beacock SM: Rabies in horses: 21 cases (1970–1990). *JAVMA* 200:1133–1137, 1992.
12. Pépin M, Blancou J, Aubert MFA: Rage expérimentale des bovins: Sensibilité, symptomes, réactions immunitaires humorales et excrétion du virus. *Ann Rech Vét* 15(3):325–333, 1984.
13. Hudson LC, Weinstock D, Jordan T, Bold-Fletcher NO: Clinical features of experimentally induced rabies in cattle and sheep. *Zentralbl Veterinarmed[B]* 43(2):85–95, 1996.
14. Chomel BB: The modern epidemiological aspects of rabies in the world. *Comp Immun Microbiol Infect Dis* 16(1):11–20, 1993.
15. Winkler WG, Jenkins SR: Raccoon rabies, in Baer GM (ed): *The Natural History of Rabies,* ed 2. Boca Raton, CRC Press, 1991, pp 326–340.
16. Fearneyhough MG, Wilson PJ, Clark KA, et al: Results of an oral rabies vaccination program for coyotes. *JAVMA.* 212:498–502, 1998.
17. Baer GM, Smith JS: Rabies in nonhematophagous bats, in Baer GM (ed): *The Natural History of Rabies,* ed 2. Boca Raton, CRC Press, 1991, pp 341–366.
18. Everard COR, Everard JD: Mongoose rabies in the Caribbean. *Ann NY Acad Sci* 653:356–366, 1992.
19. Smith JS, Seidel HD: Rabies: A new look at an old disease, in Melnick JL (ed): *Progress in Medical Virology,* vol 40. Basel, Karger, 1993, pp 82–106.

The incidence of rabies is slightly higher in colonial species of bats than in solitary species.

Rabies Exposure and Clinical Disease in Humans

Jennifer H. McQuiston, DVM, MS
James E. Childs, ScD
Viral and Rickettsial Zoonoses Branch, Division of Viral and Rickettsial Diseases
Centers for Disease Control and Prevention
Atlanta, Georgia

RABIES REMAINS A THREAT IN MANY PARTS OF THE WORLD, AND THE WORLD HEALTH ORGANIZATION (WHO) HAS ESTIMATED THAT MORE THAN 40,000 PEOPLE DIE OF RABIES EACH YEAR.[1] MOST OF THESE DEATHS ARE REPORTED IN ASIA, AFRICA, AND LATIN AMERICA, BUT OCCASIONAL HUMAN RABIES DEATHS STILL OCCUR IN THE UNITED STATES.[2-4] BECAUSE RABIES VIRUS TRANSMISSION TO HUMANS FROM WILDLIFE AND DOMESTIC ANIMALS REMAINS A POSSIBILITY IN THE UNITED STATES AND BECAUSE MANY U.S. CITIZENS TRAVEL TO AREAS WHERE CANINE RABIES IS STILL ENDEMIC, RABIES SHOULD CONTINUE TO BE CONSIDERED FOR ANY UNDIAGNOSED CASE OF ACUTE ENCEPHALITIS IN THE UNITED STATES. FURTHERMORE, PUBLIC HEALTH OFFICIALS AND MEDICAL PROFESSIONALS SHOULD BE AWARE OF THE RISKS FOR EXPOSURE TO RABIES VIRUS AND SHOULD BE ABLE TO ADVISE PERSONS WHO HAVE BEEN EXPOSED WHETHER POSTEXPOSURE PROPHYLAXIS (PEP) IS INDICATED.

The World Health Organization has estimated that more than 40,000 people die of rabies each year.

CASE REPORT

On October 12, 1997, a New Jersey man developed pain in his right shoulder and neck as well as nonspecific symptoms such as sore throat, nausea, and chills. He was initially treated as an outpatient by his local physician, but on October 14 he was admitted to the hospital because of fever, agitation, and difficulty swallowing. His illness progressed over the next several days to include hallucinations, and intubation was eventually required to protect breathing. Because rabies was suspected on the basis of clinical symptoms, several specimens were submitted to the Centers for Disease Control and Prevention on October 17 for antemortem testing. Although serum and cerebrospinal fluid were negative for antibodies to rabies virus, virus was isolated from saliva. The patient eventually died because of systemic complications. Although the patient had initially denied any contact with animals, additional information obtained from his wife revealed that he may have had contact with bats that were found in his house in July. The particular strain of rabies virus responsible for this man's death was characterized as a variant normally associated with silver-haired bats.[3]

EPIDEMIOLOGY OF HUMAN RABIES

The presentation of this case is fairly typical of many of the human rabies deaths that have

TABLE 1

Evaluating Exposures to Rabies Virus: Considerations and Treatment Guidelines

Type of Exposure	Modifying Variables	Treatment	Comments
Bite	Consider the biting species	▪ Cleanse the wound ▪ Immune globulin[a] ▪ Vaccine	Most common route of virus transmission. Exposure is usually noted, although bat bites may be difficult to detect. Even circumstantial bat exposures may warrant PEP.[b]
Nonbite ▪ Scratch ▪ Mucous membrane	Exposure to saliva or CNS material should have occurred to warrant PEP	▪ Cleanse the site ▪ Immune globulin[a] ▪ Vaccine	Uncommon route of transmission.
▪ Aerosol	Probably dependent on virus concentration in fine aerosols or droplets	▪ Immune globulin[a] ▪ Vaccine	Rare route of transmission. Cases have been described only following laboratory accidents and from caves inhabited by millions of bats.
▪ Corneal transplant	Persons dying from encephalitis or undiagnosed neurologic disease are not acceptable donors	▪ Immune globulin[a] ▪ Vaccine	Careful donor selection will lessen risks.

[a]Immune globulin is not necessary in a previously vaccinated person.
[b]PEP is recommended if there is a reasonable chance a bite from a bat may have occurred. For example, PEP should be given if a bat is found in a room with a child or a sleeping or incapacitated person.

occurred in the United States in recent years. Although human rabies is relatively rare, the incidence of cases diagnosed in this country has increased from an average of one case per year in the 1980s to an average of 3.25 cases annually in 1990 and 1997.[2–4] This increase in the incidence of human rabies deaths is striking because most of the recent cases have been caused by strains of rabies virus normally associated with bats. Humans may be at risk for rabies after exposures to bats because they may not realize they have been exposed or may not realize the risks of contracting rabies from bats.

Raccoons, skunks, bats, and foxes remain the most commonly reported species infected with rabies virus in the United States.[5] These wild animals can be responsible for the transmission of rabies virus to humans and domestic animals such as dogs, cats, and livestock.[5] Because of the close relationship between humans and domestic animals, transmission of rabies virus to humans from pets and livestock remains a concern and must be considered in the event of an exposure. In addition to the threat of contracting rabies from animals within the United States, travelers remain at risk for rabies when visiting countries where rabies is still prevalent among domestic dogs. Since 1980, 12 human rabies deaths among citizens or foreign residents in the United States have been attributed to strains of rabies virus found circulating in dog populations in foreign countries.[2]

TYPES OF EXPOSURES

There are two categories of exposures by which rabies virus may be transmitted to humans: bite exposures and nonbite exposures (Table 1). Bite exposures are the most common route for rabies virus to be transmitted. In this type of exposure, infectious saliva from an animal is inoculated directly into a fresh wound. Saliva can contain high concentrations of infectious virus, and, ac-

The incidence of

human rabies

diagnosed in the

United States has

increased from an

average of one case

per year in the

1980s to an

average of 3.25

cases annually in

the 1990s.

cordingly, this type of exposure carries the highest risk of transmission of rabies. Not all humans who are bitten by a rabid animal will develop rabies; however, all bites carry a risk of transmitting rabies and should be treated appropriately. Head and neck wounds carry the highest risk, presumably because the virus has a shorter distance to travel along peripheral nerves before reaching the central nervous system.[6] Highly innervated sites may be more readily infected, so bites to the fingers may carry a high risk as well. Hand and arm wounds carry a moderate risk, while bites to the legs carry a lesser risk.[6] Overall estimates of risk for contracting rabies associated with untreated bite wounds inflicted by rabid animals are approximately 15%, but this estimate varies, based on the site and severity of the wound.[6] Veterinarians and persons in frequent contact with wild or domestic animals obviously have an increased risk of being bitten and accordingly may be at increased risk of being infected with the rabies virus.

One complicating factor in assessing an exposure to rabies virus is an individual's awareness that a bite has occurred. Typically, bites received from large terrestrial carnivores such as skunks, raccoons, or dogs are noticed, and appropriate actions are taken for treatment. Bites from bats, however, may be more difficult to detect. Many recent cases of human rabies associated with variants of rabies virus maintained by bats involved persons who either did not notice, recall, or appreciate that an exposing event had occurred.[2] Given the rarity of rabies virus transmission by events other than bite exposures, an unnoticed or unappreciated bat bite was the most likely route of transmission among these individuals.

Nonbite exposures are a less important route of transmission and occur infrequently in nature. Because saliva and material from the central nervous system may be infectious, contamination of scratches, open wounds, or mucous membranes with these substances could result in transmission of rabies virus. However, there are few validated examples of such cases, and the risk of developing rabies after this type of exposure if left untreated is estimated to be only approximately 0.1%.[6] Rabies virus has been isolated from respiratory secretions and tears of humans, although at lower levels than saliva, so these fluids may carry a lesser risk for virus transmission.[7] Exposure to human or animal blood, feces, or unconcentrated urine does not pose a risk for transmission of rabies, as virus is not found in these substances.[7,8] Transplacental and perinatal transmission of rabies virus among some animals and humans has been reported and should be considered a possibility in certain situations.[9–12] Because the clinical signs of rabies in domestic animals may be quite variable, veterinarians who are suspicious of rabies in an animal should wear gloves when performing oral or postmortem examinations.

Additional types of nonbite exposures have rarely been documented. Aerosolized rabies virus suspended in fine droplets of saliva or respiratory fluids has been implicated in two human deaths associated with bat caves inhabited by millions of Mexican free-tailed bats,[13,14] and aerosol transmission is also suspected in two laboratory accidents.[15,16] Transmission of rabies virus has also occurred following corneal transplants from donors with undiagnosed rabies; as a result, the Eye Bank Association of America has adopted standards stating that persons dying from encephalitis or undiagnosed neurologic disease are not acceptable donors.[17–22] Recently, possible transmission of rabies virus between a mother and child was reported in Ethiopia when the only reported contact was kissing.[10] In general, these cases are considered isolated incidents.

DECIDING WHEN TO ADMINISTER PEP

Although the mortality rate for persons showing clinical symptoms of rabies is near-

Many recent cases of human rabies associated with variants of rabies virus maintained by bats involved persons who either did not notice, recall, or appreciate that an exposing event had occurred.

ly 100%, human rabies is a preventable disease even after exposure has occurred. PEP consisting of human rabies immune globulin and five doses of vaccine is widely available in the United States, and correct and timely administration provides complete protection against the development of clinical rabies in humans. Determining whether PEP is needed can be a difficult task, and each situation should be assessed on an individual basis. State and local health officials can advise persons of their risks and make recommendations for treatment, but the decision to actually administer PEP lies with the patient and the patient's physician. The Advisory Committee on Immunization Practices (ACIP) has issued recommendations regarding rabies prevention, and physicians and medical professionals should follow these guidelines when deciding whether PEP is needed.[23] In most cases, a bite from a rabid or presumed rabid animal must have occurred, or infectious material must have come in contact with an open wound or mucous membrane for PEP to be warranted. In addition, the type of animal involved in the exposure and whether it is available for observation or immediate euthanasia and testing for rabies virus will influence the decision on PEP.

In the United States, wild carnivores such as raccoons, skunks, foxes, bobcats, and coyotes may have a high risk of rabies and should be considered potentially rabid until proved otherwise.[23] Although these animals are considered most likely to be infected with rabies virus in certain geographic locations within the United States,[5] they have the potential to contract the virus from other species and transmit rabies in any setting. Ideally, any wild carnivore that exposes a human should be euthanized and its brain should be tested for the presence of rabies virus. Exposed persons should begin PEP immediately and discontinue vaccinations only if the animal tests negative.[23] In most situations, an animal that cannot be captured is assumed to be rabid, and PEP

should be administered to the exposed person immediately.[23]

Bats should be considered rabid until shown otherwise through laboratory testing, regardless of the geographic location.[23] Rabid bats have been reported from each state within the continental United States, and a rabid bat was identified in Hawaii following translocation by boat from the mainland.[24] Because bites from insectivorous bats may be difficult to detect, each situation should be assessed carefully. Persons who handle bats with their bare hands may not be able to rule out the possibility of a bat bite. Similarly, if a bat is found in a room with a sleeping or incapacitated individual or a young child, it may be assumed that an exposure could have occurred even if there is no physical evidence of a bite or scratch. Ideally, the bat should be safely captured and tested for rabies. PEP should be started immediately, but it may be discontinued if the bat tests negative for rabies.[23] If the bat is not available for testing, it should be assumed to be rabid and PEP should be administered immediately to the exposed person.[23]

In the United States, bites from vaccinated domestic carnivores are considered to carry a lower risk of rabies virus transmission. Healthy dogs, cats, and ferrets that expose a person through a bite or saliva contact may be observed for 10 days to see if they develop clinical signs of rabies.[8] This observation period is necessary even if the animal is currently vaccinated against rabies, because occasional vaccine failures have been documented in dogs and cats.[25, 26] Exposed persons do not need to begin PEP unless the animal becomes sick or dies from rabies during this observation period.[23] If the animal becomes ill or dies, it should be tested for rabies, and exposed persons should begin PEP immediately. If the animal is subsequently shown to be negative for the presence of rabies virus through laboratory tests, PEP can be discontinued.[23] If the dog, cat, or ferret is not available for testing or observation, public health officials should be consulted to determine PEP recommendations. If the attack was unprovoked or if the animal was a stray with an unknown vaccination history, PEP should be administered.

In contrast to carnivores and bats, exposures to wild animals such as rodents (mice, rats, and squirrels), ungulates (deer), and lagomorphs (rabbits and hares) carry a very low risk for rabies, and PEP is generally not recommended. However, rabies is occasionally documented in these species,[5] and in some cases rabies testing or PEP administration may be recommended at the discretion of health officials if the animal was sick or behaving strangely. In particular, reports of rabies in woodchucks (also known as groundhogs) and beavers have increased in recent years,[27] and PEP may occasionally be indicated following exposures to these animals. Domestic herbivores such as horses, sheep, goats, and pigs are assumed to have a low risk for rabies, although cattle are reported rabid at a frequency similar to that in dogs.[5] Again, each situation should be considered on an individual basis, and PEP may be recommended at the discretion of local health officials.

Although an observation period of 10 days may be initiated following an exposure from a dog, cat, or ferret,[8] observation periods are not recommended following exposures from other animals. The 10-day observation period in dogs, cats, and ferrets is based on laboratory data demonstrating that virus may be shed in saliva for a few days before the development of clinical signs of rabies in these species.[8] However, definitive studies on viral shedding have not been conducted for other species, and appropriate observation periods and typical clinical signs have not been established. Therefore, the decision to administer PEP following an exposure to a wild animal or domestic herbivore should be based on the guidelines already described rather than on arbitrary observation periods.

Persons traveling in foreign countries should be aware of risks associated with bites from dogs and, in some instances, from native wildlife. In many countries, dogs should be considered rabid unless proved otherwise, and PEP should be sought in the event of an exposure. WHO provides information on reported rabies cases from many countries, and some countries are considered "rabies-free." Decisions to administer PEP may depend on the prevalence of rabies in a given area.

Although human-to-human transmission of rabies virus is poorly documented, it remains a possibility. Therefore, PEP may be recommended for persons who have had contact with a human rabies case. While a bite exposure is unlikely between humans, contact of saliva with open wounds or mucous membranes is possible. Generally, healthcare personnel and close family members who may have been exposed to saliva, tears, or respiratory fluids from the patient should be evaluated, and PEP should be administered to those with documented exposures.[7]

DECIDING WHEN PREEXPOSURE VACCINATION IS WARRANTED

Persons who may be more likely to be exposed to rabies virus during occupational or recreational activities should consider receiving the preexposure vaccination series (Table 2). Preexposure vaccination simplifies the administration of PEP and may provide a measure of protection in the event that a true exposure is not realized.[23] Persons who should consider preexposure vaccination include veterinarians and animal control officers, mammologists, spelunkers and other persons who may spend time in caves, and workers who may encounter rabies virus in a laboratory setting. In addition, persons traveling or living in other countries where canine rabies is prevalent should consider receiving the preexposure vaccination series. A history of preexposure vaccination, however, does not eliminate the need for appropriate wound treatment

In many countries, dogs should be considered rabid unless proved otherwise.

TABLE 2
Recommendations for Rabies Vaccination by Type of Exposure

Type of Exposure	Recommendations
Continuous (laboratory workers)	Preexposure vaccination, titer checks every 6 months; boosters recommended if titer falls below 1:5 on a rapid fluorescent focus inhibition test (RFFIT); abbreviated PEP schedule given as needed in the event of an exposure
Episodic (veterinarians, animal control officers, spelunkers, wildlife handlers)	Preexposure vaccination; abbreviated PEP schedule given in the event of an exposure
Sporadic/Unpredictable (general public)	PEP given only in the event of an exposure to a rabid or presumed rabid animal
Foreign travel to countries with endemic canine rabies	Preexposure vaccination may be warranted; PEP given according to ACIP guidelines in the event of an exposure to a rabid or presumed rabid animal

and additional vaccinations as recommended by the ACIP.

PROPHYLAXIS FOLLOWING A RABIES EXPOSURE

Once an exposure has occurred, it is very important to follow the correct steps for PEP. Furthermore, PEP should be initiated regardless of how much time may have elapsed since the exposure. Appropriate PEP includes wound cleansing, administration of human rabies immune globulin for previously unvaccinated individuals, and vaccination with an approved cell culture–derived vaccine. The wound or exposed area should be washed thoroughly with soap and water, and if possible an antiseptic should be applied.[23] Cleansing wounds in this manner will dramatically decrease the chance of developing rabies.[28]

In the United States, immune globulin and approved cell culture–derived vaccines should be administered in accordance with guidelines issued by the ACIP.[23] The protocol presented by WHO offers different treatment options,[1] but these options are not recognized by the ACIP. The ACIP guidelines do not advocate changing treatment options based on the severity of the exposure or the location of the wound on the body and state that all exposures should be treated according to uniform guidelines. Although current WHO recommendations describe the use of alternate vaccination schedules for PEP,[1] these variations of protocol are not recommended by the ACIP. In addition, the ACIP does not recommend vaccination with neural tissue–derived vaccines because of the risk of adverse side effects.[23] Persons in foreign countries should be especially careful when seeking PEP and should make every effort to receive cell culture–derived rabies vaccine and human rabies immune globulin as recommended by the ACIP.[23]

CLINICAL RABIES IN HUMANS

The incubation period for rabies in humans is quite variable, with most persons developing clinical symptoms within several weeks to several months following exposure. However, incubation periods in humans as long as 6 years after the last possible exposure have been documented.[29] The incubation period is dependent on many factors, including the site of the inoculation, the dose of rabies virus, and the length of time the virus may spend in nonneuronal tissues. Infectious virus may be shed in the saliva for a brief time near the end of the incubation period and before the onset of clinical symptoms. Therefore, when potential exposures are assessed following a positive diagnosis of rabies in a human, persons who may have had exposure to the patient for a period preceding the diagnosis are often given PEP.

Human rabies classically begins with a prodromal syndrome consisting of nonspecific symptoms. The prodromal syndrome correlates to the early presence of the virus in the central nervous system and may present with vague flulike or gastrointestinal symptoms. Many persons report headache, malaise, insomnia, or anxiety; in addition, pain or paresthesia may be reported near the site of the original bite.[6,30] The length of the prodromal period varies from 2 to 7 days, and many persons seek repeated medical care during this time. Most individuals are initially treated as outpatients because of the vague nature of the clinical symptoms,[2] although hospitalization eventually occurs as the patient develops symptoms of nervous system involvement. Two main categories of neurologic symptoms may be present; they are classically referred to as "furious" rabies and "dumb" or paralytic rabies.[30–32]

Paralytic rabies is the less common form of human rabies, occurring in an estimated 20% of cases, and presents mainly with symptoms of muscle spasms and ascending paralysis that may resemble Guillain-Barré syndrome.[6,30–32] This form of rabies may be misdiagnosed because of the lack of classic symptoms such as hydrophobia and behavioral changes. Paralytic rabies often has a longer clinical course than the furious form but is still fatal because of respiratory paralysis and complications.

The majority of human rabies cases develop clinical symptoms of furious rabies, although symptoms of paralytic rabies may occur near the end of illness. Virus localization in the limbic system of the brain results in behavioral changes that may be characterized by symptoms such as hyperactivity, hallucinations, and mood swings.[30–32] Various clinical symptoms attributable to stimulation of the autonomic nervous system may be observed, such as excessive salivation, sweating, and miosis.[30] Seizures or muscle fasciculations may occur in some patients, and classic symptoms of hydrophobia may be present in up to 50% of patients.[32] Hydrophobia may be caused by pharyngeal spasms that are induced when the patient attempts to swallow fluids, although the psychological effects of rabies virus infection may also contribute to the patient's fear of swallowing. Patients may become belligerent or violent, and some require sedation. Nervous system excitement may be triggered by auditory or visual stimulation and may occur unexpectedly between periods when the patient appears aware of his or her surroundings. The clinical symptoms progress over a course of several days, eventually leading to coma and death.

Complications of both forms of rabies are numerous and often contribute directly to the patient's death. Fluctuating body temperatures are common and result from the influence of rabies virus on the thermoregulatory center in the hypothalamus.[30] Symptoms of polyuria due to diabetes insipidus may result from the influence of rabies virus on the pituitary gland,[6,30] and severe dehydration is a common complication. Paralysis of respiratory muscles can result in hypoxia and asphyxiation if mechanical ventilation is not available, and bronchopneumonia may be a complication due to respiratory collapse.[30] Cardiovascular complications are common and involve ventricular arrhythmias and tachycardia; in addition to being caused by hypoxia, a primary rabies myocarditis may contribute to these findings.[31,32] Cerebral hypoxia due to respiratory compromise can cause increased intracranial pressure, which can lead to seizures and coma.[6,30]

Laboratory findings may indicate a nonspecific infectious cause. The peripheral white blood cell count is often elevated,[30] and serum chemistries may show numerous

If rabies is suspected in a human, antemortem tests are available that may aid in a diagnosis.

Medical therapy

such as use of

antiviral agents

has not proved

effective in the

treatment of

rabies infection.

abnormalities that reflect the systemic complications already listed. If rabies is suspected in a human, antemortem tests are available that may aid in a diagnosis. Screening for rabies atigen using nuchal skin biopsies is more sensitive than using corneal impressions and can be a useful diagnostic tool.[2] Rising serum antibody titers may be diagnostic, although antibodies may not be present early in the course of disease; in addition, the presence of antibodies against rabies virus in cerebrospinal fluid is indicative of active infection. Newer diagnostic techniques, such as reverse transcriptase polymerase chain reaction (RT-PCR), have also proved useful for demonstrating the presence of rabies virus in various tissues. However, a negative antemortem result does not completely rule out rabies, because the disease is most reliably confirmed after death.

Reports of human rabies deaths in the United States are unusual. However, some recent reports of infection have been based solely on postmortem examination of tissues, and the possibility exists that some cases could be missed, particularly when rabies is not suspected before the death of the patient. Between 1980 and 1997, an antemortem diagnosis of rabies was considered in only 20 of 32 human rabies cases, and the presence of "classic" clinical symptoms, such as hydrophobia or aerophobia, was significantly associated with a correct diagnosis.[2] It is worth noting that modern medical treatment for persons with behavioral changes such as those that might be manifested early in rabies virus infection often involves the use of sedatives, which may in fact mask some "classic" behaviors.

With few exceptions, rabies is a fatal illness, and without significant supportive measures death usually occurs within several days of the onset of clinical symptoms. Medical therapy such as use of antiviral agents has not proved effective in the treatment of rabies infection. Medical support and mechanical ventilation may prolong survival times for longer periods, but pa-

tients are usually comatose during this time. Accounts of recovery following human rabies infection are rare, and neurologic sequelae usually result.[16,33,34]

SUMMARY

Although rabies is a preventable illness, correct recognition of an exposure and appropriate administration of PEP are essential for the prevention of human rabies deaths. The recommendations from the ACIP can guide medical professionals as they make decisions regarding the need for PEP. Although human rabies is a rare illness in the United States, it should continue to be a differential diagnosis for any case of acute progressive encephalitis.

REFERENCES

1. World Health Organization: *WHO Expert Committee on Rabies, 8th Report.* 824:1–84, 1992.
2. Noah DL, Drenzek CL, Smith JS, et al: Epidemiology of human rabies in the United States, 1980 to 1996. *Ann Intern Med* 128:922–930, 1998.
3. Centers for Disease Control and Prevention: Human rabies—Texas and New Jersey, 1997. *MMWR Morb Mortal Wkly Rep* 47:1–5, 1998.
4. Centers for Disease Control and Prevention: Human rabies—Montana and Washington, 1997. *MMWR Morb Mortal Wkly Rep* 44:770–774, 1997.
5. Krebs JW, Smith JS, Rupprecht CE, Childs JE: Rabies surveillance in the United States during 1996. *JAVMA* 211:1525–1539, 1997.
6. Hattwick MAW: Human rabies. *Public Health Rev* 3:229–274, 1974.
7. Helmick CG, Tauxe RV, Vernon AA: Is there a risk to contacts of patients with rabies? *Rev Infect Dis* 9:511–518, 1987.
8. Compendium of Animal Rabies Control, 1998. *JAVMA* 212:213–217, 1998.
9. Sipahioglu U, Alpaut S: Transplacental rabies in humans. *Mikrobiyol Bul* 19:95–99, 1985.
10. Fekadu M, Endeshaw T, Alemu W, et al: Possible human-to-human transmission of rabies in Ethiopia. *Ethiop Med J* 34:123–127, 1996.
11. Howard DR: Transplacental transmission of rabies virus from a naturally infected skunk. *Am J Vet Res* 42:691–692, 1981.
12. Martell MA, Montes FC, Alcocer R: Transplacental transmission of bovine rabies after natural infection. *J Infect Dis* 127:291–293, 1973.
13. Constantine DG: Rabies transmission by nonbite route. *Public Health Rep* 77:287–289, 1962.
14. Winkler WG: Airborne rabies virus isolation. *Bull Wildl Dis Assoc* 4:37–40, 1968.
15. Conomy JP, Leibovitz A, McCombs W, Stinson J: Airborne rabies encephalitis: Demonstration of rabies virus in the human central nervous system. *Neurology* 27:67–69, 1977.

16. Centers for Disease Control: Rabies in a laboratory worker—New York. *MMWR Morb Mortal Wkly Rep* 26:183–184, 1977.

17. Gode GR, Bhinde NK: Two rabies deaths after corneal grafts from one donor. *Lancet* 2:791, 1988.

18. Centers for Disease Control: Human-to-human transmission of rabies via a corneal transplant—France. *MMWR Morb Mortal Wkly Rep* 29:25–26, 1980.

19. Houff SA, Burton RC, Wilson RW, et al: Human-to-human transmission of rabies virus by corneal transplant. *N Engl J Med* 300:603–604, 1979.

20. World Health Organization: Two rabies cases following corneal transplantation. *Weekly Epidemiol Rec* 69:330, 1994.

21. Javadi MA, Fayaz A, Mirdehghan SA, Ainollahi B: Transmission of rabies by corneal graft. *Cornea* 15:431–433, 1996.

22. Eye Bank Association of America: *Eye Bank Association of America Medical Standards.* Section D1:8–13, 1997.

23. Centers for Disease Control and Prevention: Human Rabies Prevention--United States, 1999: Recommendations of the Advisory Committee on Immunization Practices (ACIP). *MMWR Morb Mortal Wkly Rep* RR-1:1–21, 1999.

24. Krebs JW, Holman RC, Hines U, et al: Rabies surveillance in the United States during 1991. *JAVMA* 201:1836–1848, 1992.

25. Eng TR, Fishbein DB: Epidemiologic factors, clinical findings, and vaccination status of rabies in cats and dogs in the United States in 1988. *JAVMA* 197:201–209, 1990.

26. Clark KA, Wilson PJ: Postexposure rabies prophylaxis and preexposure rabies vaccination failure in domestic animals. *JAVMA* 208:1827–1830, 1996.

27. Childs JE, Colby L, Krebs JW, et al: Surveillance and spatiotemporal associations of rabies in rodents and lagomorphs in the United States, 1985–1994. *J Wildl Dis* 33:20–27, 1997.

28. Dean DJ, Baer GM, Thompson WR: Studies on the local treatment of rabies-infected wounds. *Bull World Health Organ* 28:477–486, 1963.

29. Smith JS, Fishbein DB, Rupprecht CE, Clark K: Unexplained rabies in three immigrants in the United States. *New Engl J Med* 324:205–211, 1991.

30. Warrell DA: The clinical picture of rabies in man. *Trans R Soc Trop Med Hyg* 70:188–195, 1976.

31. Hemachudha T: Human rabies: Clinical aspects, pathogenesis, and potential therapy. *Curr Top Microbiol Immunol* 187:121–143, 1994.

32. Mrak RE, Young L: Rabies encephalitis in humans: Pathology, pathogenesis, and pathophysiology. *J Neuropathol Exp Neurol* 53:1–10, 1994.

33. Hattwick MAW, Weis TT, Stechschulte CJ, et al: Recovery from rabies: A case report. *Ann Intern Med* 76:931–942, 1972.

34. Alvarez LH, Fajardo RV, Lopez EM, et al: Partial recovery from rabies in a nine-year-old boy. *Pediatr Infect Dis J* 13:1154–1155, 1994.

Preexposure Rabies Immunoprophylaxis

David W. Dreesen, DVM, MPVM
Diplomate ACVPM
Private Consultant, Lida Corporation
Winterville, Georgia

Once the signs of rabies occur in warm-blooded animals, the disease is nearly always fatal.

ALTHOUGH THERE IS EVIDENCE THAT, IN RARE INSTANCES, ANIMALS WITH RABIES MAY RECOVER, ONE SHOULD CONSIDER, ESPECIALLY IN HUMANS, THAT ONCE THE SIGNS OF RABIES OCCUR IN WARM-BLOODED ANIMALS, THE DISEASE IS NEARLY ALWAYS FATAL.[1,2] IN 1995, THE WORLD HEALTH ORGANIZATION REPORTED MORE THAN 40,000 HUMAN DEATHS WORLDWIDE DUE TO RABIES. PERHAPS ANOTHER 10,000 TO 15,000 DEATHS GO UNREPORTED.[3] THE VAST MAJORITY OF THESE DEATHS OCCUR IN REGIONS OF THE WORLD WHERE CANINE RABIES IS ENDEMIC. FREE-RUNNING AND FERAL DOGS, AS WELL AS UNVACCINATED PET DOGS, IN SUCH REGIONS CONSTITUTE A VIRTUAL RESERVOIR FOR THE RABIES VIRUS. A GREAT NUMBER OF THESE HUMAN RABIES DEATHS COULD PROBABLY BE PREVENTED BY PROPER IMMUNIZATION OF DOGS AGAINST THIS DREAD DISEASE. THE EPIDEMIOLOGIC EVIDENCE SHOWS THAT WHERE CANINE RABIES VACCINATION IS A ROUTINE MATTER, ALONG WITH FUNCTIONAL ANIMAL CONTROL PROGRAMS, RABIES DEATHS ATTRIBUTABLE TO DOG BITES ARE RARE EVENTS.[4] IN ADDITION, PERSONS WHO ARE AT HIGH RISK FOR RABIES, SUCH AS THOSE IN RESEARCH LABORATORIES WORKING WITH THE VIRUS, ANIMAL CONTROL PERSONNEL, VETERINARIANS AND THEIR ANIMAL-HANDLING STAFF, SPELUNKERS, AT-RISK PERSONS TRAVELING TO RABIES-ENZOOTIC AREAS, AND OTHERS CAN BE IMMUNIZED, THUS REDUCING THEIR RISK FOR THE DISEASE.[5-7] RABIES VACCINATION OF DOGS, CATS, AND OTHER DOMESTIC ANIMALS IS ALSO OF PRIME IMPORTANCE TO PRODUCE A "BUFFER ZONE" OF VACCINATED ANIMALS BETWEEN WILD ANIMAL SPECIES AND HUMANS, AS WELL AS TO LOWER THE ECONOMIC LOSSES OF FOOD ANIMALS, ESPECIALLY CATTLE, DUE TO RABIES DEATHS. ORAL RABIES VACCINE PROGRAMS TARGETED TOWARD CERTAIN WILDLIFE SPECIES HAVE ALSO BECOME AN IMPORTANT FACTOR IN OUR EFFORTS TO INTERRUPT THE TRANSMISSION CYCLE OF RABIES.[8]

PREEXPOSURE RABIES PROPHYLAXIS FOR HUMANS

Preexposure prophylaxis (PrEP) should be made available to persons at risk for exposure to the virus through either known or inapparent exposure to the virus. The criteria for those who should receive PrEP, based on risk, are outlined in Table 1[6] and have been reviewed in *The Nat-*

TABLE 1
Rabies Preexposure Prophylaxis Guide—United States, 1999

Risk Category	Nature of Risk	Typical Populations	Preexposure Recommendations[a]
Continuous	Virus present continuously, often in high concentrations; specific exposures likely to go unrecognized; bite, nonbite, or aerosol exposure	Rabies research laboratory workers,[a] rabies biologics production workers	Primary course; serologic testing every 6 months; booster vaccination if antibody titer is below acceptable level[b]
Frequent	Exposure usually episodic, with source recognized, but exposure also might be unrecognized; bite, nonbite, or aerosol exposure	Rabies diagnostic laboratory workers,[a] spelunkers, veterinarians and staff, animal-control and wildlife workers in rabies-enzootic areas	Primary course; serologic testing every 2 years; booster vaccination if antibody titer is below acceptable level[b]
Infrequent (greater than population at large)	Exposure nearly always episodic with source recognized; bite or nonbite exposure	Veterinarians, animal-control and wildlife workers in areas with low rabies rates; veterinary students; travelers visiting areas where rabies is enzootic and immediate access to appropriate medical care including biologics is limited	Primary course; no serologic testing or booster vaccination
Rare (population at large)	Exposure always episodic with source recognized; bite or nonbite exposure	U.S. population at large, including persons in rabies-epizootic areas	No vaccination necessary

[a]Judgment of relative risk and extra monitoring of vaccination status of laboratory workers are the responsibilities of the laboratory supervisor.
[b]Minimum acceptable antibody level is complete virus neutralization at a 1:5 serum dilution by the rapid fluorescent focus inhibition test. A booster dose should be administered if the titer falls below this level.

ural History of Rabies, second edition.[7] The efficacy of PrEP has been well demonstrated in animal challenge studies and from evidence based on humoral response in humans to the vaccines in numerous controlled clinical trials.

According to the recommendations of the Advisory Committee on Immunization Practices (ACIP) of the U.S. Public Health Service, one dose each of PrEP should be administered on days 0, 7, and 28 by either the intramuscular (IM) route or the intradermal (ID) route (depending on the vaccine) in the upper deltoid region of the arm.[6] However, persons at continuous risk of rabies virus (Table 1) should receive the vaccine via the IM route of administration only. The route of administration should not be mixed during the three-dose series.[6] Vaccines approved by the Food and Drug Administration (FDA) for PrEP use in the United States are shown in Table 2.

It is essential that the rabies vaccine be administered exactly according to package insert instructions. ID vaccinations must be given by personnel experienced in administering ID vaccinations. A good "bleb" or "wheal" must be formed at the site of the ID vaccination. Should this not occur and the vaccine be delivered subcutaneously (SC), it is recommended that the dose be readministered.[9–11] Rabies neutralizing anti-

Persons at continuous risk of rabies virus should receive the vaccine via the IM route of administration only.

TABLE 2
Vaccines Approved for PrEP Use in the United States

Imovax® Rabies—for IM use only; Imovax® Rabies I.D.—for ID use only
   Human diploid cell culture vaccines
   Manufactured by Pasteur Mérieux Connaught Vaccines and Serums, Lyon, France
   Distributed in the United States by Pasteur Mérieux Connaught, Swiftwater, PA

RabAvert®—for IM use only
   A purified chick embryo cell culture vaccine
   Manufactured by Chiron Behring GmhH & Co., Marburg, Germany
   Distributed in the United States by Chiron Vaccines, Inc., Emeryville, CA

Most individuals

report few or no

adverse reactions

to PrEP

vaccinations with

the exception of

local pain at the

site of the

injection.

body titer reaches a peak level at approximately 49 days after the first dose of vaccine.[12,13] Antibody gradually declines in a characteristic half-life over time, depending on the individual and the route of administration, that is, IM or ID.[14] Although antibody response does not always equate to protection, guidelines for an adequate response as determined by the rapid fluorescent focus inhibition test is considered to be $\geq$1:5 (0.5 international units).[6] The term "adequate" is used rather than "protective," as no challenge studies can be ethically conducted on humans following PrEP. The ACIP recommends that an antibody titer be determined 2 years after the last dose (6 months for those in the continuous-risk group) and a single IM or ID booster dose be administered if titer is <1:5.[6]

Most individuals report few or no adverse reactions to PrEP vaccinations with the exception of local pain at the site of the injection, which is to be expected. A small percentage of individuals (up to 6%) who receive either Imovax® Rabies or Imovax® Rabies I.D. (human diploid cell [Pasteur Mérieux Connaught Vaccines and Serums]) as a primary series and then subsequently receive a booster dose of human diploid cell vaccine (IM or ID) may develop a type III hypersensitivity reaction. The illness is characterized by onset 2 to 21 days postbooster with a generalized urticaria and may also include nausea and malaise. The

signs are transitory and not life-threatening.[15,16]

Persons who have received a three-dose series of a cell culture vaccine within the past 2 to 3 years or who have a rabies-neutralizing antibody titer of $\geq$1:5 and are exposed to the virus require only two doses of a licensed rabies vaccine for postexposure prophylaxis, one dose each IM in the deltoid region on days 0 and 3.[6] Rabies immune globulin is contraindicated. Immediate and thorough local wound therapy is an essential part of any rabies postexposure therapy. Exposures involving laboratory personnel should be handled on a case-by-case basis.

PREEXPOSURE PROPHYLAXIS FOR ANIMALS

On page 79 of this publication is the *Compendium of Animal Rabies Control, 1999.* This *Compendium* is the result of a yearly report of the Compendium Committee of the National Association of State Public Health Veterinarians (NASPHV) and is recognized as the definitive guideline for animal rabies control in the United States. It is published annually, usually in January, in the *Journal of the American Veterinary Medical Association.*[17]

Dogs, Cats, and Ferrets

Effective vaccination and control programs targeted at canines in the United States have substantially reduced rabies in this population. From yearly reports of upwards of 7,000 rabies cases in dogs in the 1940s and early 1950s to fewer than 130 cases annually at present demonstrates the effectiveness of the rabies vaccines currently on the market.[4] From an epidemiologic point of view, the effectiveness of dog vaccination and control programs can also be seen by comparing trends noted in dog rabies cases to the recent increase in reported cat rabies cases.[4,8] As the raccoon epidemic moved through the middle Atlantic and northeastern United States, the number of cases of cat rabies increased substantially while the cases of canine rabies remained essentially the same, although at times there was a noticeable increase in cases of rabies in dogs in the early months of an outbreak of rabies in the local raccoon population. Currently (1997), more cases of rabies in cats (300) than in dogs (126) are reported annually in the United States.[4] This increase in cat rabies cases in the face of the raccoon outbreak in the eastern regions of the United States, while dog cases remained substantially unchanged or decreasing, reflects the vaccine rabies status of the two populations as well as the number of feral animals in the two populations.[19,20] In a study based on 1988 data, only 43% of rabid cats were owned pets.[19] The need for cat rabies vaccinations and feral population control cannot be emphasized enough.

In 1998 after extensive research studies into the pathogenicity of rabies in ferrets at the Centers for Disease Control and Prevention (CDC)[21] and the reports of the efficacy of vaccine trials in this species, the Compendium Committee recommended use of the United States Department of Agriculture (USDA)–approved Imrab® 3 rabies vaccine (Merial) for vaccination of ferrets against rabies.[18] Through September 1998, only 14 of 103 ferrets challenged with one of six rabies virus variants and having the virus in their brains also had virus in the salivary glands. Incubation periods ranged from 11 to 96 days (M. Niezgoda, CDC, personal communication). Further, the Compendium Committee recommended that ferrets be treated in the same manner as cats and dogs regarding rabies preexposure vaccination and management.

All animal rabies vaccines currently licensed must protect at least 87% of those vaccinated against challenge in a controlled clinical trial, while at least 80% of nonvaccinates should develop rabies.[22] The Compendium of Animal Rabies Control, 1999,[17] gives current vaccination recommendations.

The most common postvaccinal nonneurologic complications are soreness, lameness, and regional lymphadenomegaly in the limb in which the vaccine was injected. Fever and systemic signs, including anaphylaxis, have been observed with the use of tissue culture vaccines because of their higher antigenic mass and use of adjuvants. Focal cutaneous vasculitis and granulomas have been noted 3 to 6 months after vaccination.[23] Although postvaccinal sarcomas may develop in both dogs and cats, they are more common in cats.[23] Sarcomas may develop when the inflammatory reactions are sustained, some of which may develop months to years later.[24,25] These sarcomas are often aggressive and invasive.[23] Other postvaccinal adverse reactions have been described.

Wolf Hybrids

There are no rabies vaccines licensed for use in wolf hybrids, and most states do not allow these animals to be legally owned by private citizens. However, it is possible that tens of thousands of these animals are in private ownership and that many veterinarians will vaccinate these animals with rabies vaccines. The issue of rabies vaccination for wolf hybrids and other domestic animals crossbred with wild species has yet to be resolved. Although both dogs and wolves belong to the family Canidae, taxonomic issues have been raised as to the evolution of dogs and wolves and their genetic closeness. Various reports suggest that dogs and gray

Currently, more cases of rabies in cats than in dogs are reported annually in the United States.

wolves are each other's closest relative, that dogs are recently descended from wolves, and that the major difference in morphology between the two is the result of human selection. Thus, it may be rightly asked why a vaccine developed for domestic dogs would not be effective for wolves or wolf hybrids. It is well known that animals respond differently to various medications; thus, a different level of antigenic value of the vaccine might be required for wolf hybrids. From a biological point of view, there is little reason to believe that canine vaccines would not protect wolf hybrids; however, as noted by the 1998 Compendium of Animal Rabies Committee, "There is little scientific data on whether rabies vaccine will protect wolf hybrids or how long these animals incubate rabies or shed virus prior to recognizable signs."[18] These were the same concerns expressed by this Compendium Committee for ferrets until controlled studies resolved the issues[21] and the ferret was added to the list of species recommended by the Compendium Committee to be vaccinated against rabies and managed in the same manner as dogs and cats, for exposures to and by the animal.[18]

In a letter to state public health veterinarians, state epidemiologists, and state veterinarians that accompanied the *Compendium of Animal Rabies Control, 1998,* it was noted that a meeting of taxonomists and others in April 1996 concluded that rabies vaccines for dogs would probably protect wolves and their hybrids. The concern was for the safety of other vaccines (distemper, adenovirus type 2, parvovirus, leptospirosis, coronavirus, etc.) in wolves and wolf hybrids, especially the modified live vaccines (MLVs). If the USDA expands a vaccine label to include rabies, it is required to do the same for the other vaccines. USDA has requested data on the safety of all vaccines, especially the MLVs, in wolves and wolf hybrids so that they can evaluate the safety information, as available. This agency has stated that if field studies from accumulated

data show that the MLVs are equally safe for hybrids as for dogs, all dog vaccines will be approved for use in hybrids. There has been at least one report in the literature of rabies vaccine failure in a wolf-dog hybrid.

Cattle, Sheep, and Horses

Similar to other domestic species, the number of reported cases of rabies in cattle has declined from nearly 1,000 per year in the mid-1950s to fewer than 150 per year.[4] Much of this decrease can be attributed to the decrease in dog rabies cases. Currently, most cases of cattle rabies occur in areas where the disease is endemic in skunks. Iowa (37) and North Dakota (16) reported 40% of all cattle rabies cases (131) in the United States in 1996.[4] Rabies in horses has remained relatively constant over the last 20 years, with approximately 45 to 60 reported cases per year, most of these occurring also in the areas where skunk rabies is endemic.[4,26] Rabies in sheep is rarely reported. This may be due to less exposure risk or to the fact that an attack by a rabid dog(s) or wild animals such as foxes and coyotes usually results in the death of the sheep or lamb and a laboratory confirmation is not requested.

PrEP is recommended for valuable cattle and horses in areas where rabies is epidemic or endemic in wild animal species.[17] Although these species are not considered to be important in the transmission cycle of the disease, their death can be a considerable economic or sentimental loss. The *Compendium of Animal Rabies Control, 1999,* lists four rabies vaccines licensed for cattle and five for sheep and horses.[17] With but two exceptions, the animal should be vaccinated at 1 year of age and then annually, with either a 1.0- or 2.0-ml dose, administered SC or IM, depending on the vaccine. The exceptions: Merial's Imrab 3 and Imrab® Bovine Plus vaccines are licensed for use in sheep on a triennial basis after an initial 2.0-ml dose at 3 months and a booster at 1 year.

The management of horses and livestock

exposed to rabies virus is covered in the *Compendium of Animal Rabies Control, 1999,* Part III, B 5b.[17]

Wildlife and Zoological Animals

There are no licensed parenteral rabies vaccines approved for use in wild or zoo-kept wild animals.[17] However, in 1983 an effective oral vaccine was developed using the rabies glycoprotein and a live vaccinia virus as a vector.[27] Following safety field trials targeted toward raccoons in 1990 on Parramore Island, VA, and in 1991 in central Pennsylvania, the vaccine, Raboral™ (Merial), was released for efficacy studies in raccoons in New Jersey during 1992 and in Cape Cod, MA, in 1994.[8] The success of these safety and efficacy trials led to the first use of the vaccine for control of endemic raccoon rabies in Albany and Rensselaer counties in New York and elsewhere in the state. New York currently has ongoing programs in the Niagara–St. Lawrence River area, Lake Erie region, and along the Vermont border. Oral rabies vaccine programs directed at raccoons have also been implemented in Pinellas County, FL; Cape Cod, MA; and Cape May, NJ.[8] Although oral rabies vaccination of raccoons shows some promise for control of rabies in this species in limited outbreak areas, its overall feasibility is still somewhat questionable. Primary among several factors that cause problems in control programs is the extensive geographic area affected with raccoon rabies (1,000,000 km²),[8] as well as the cost of continuing programs over several years. However, the oral rabies vaccine program in Ohio has had considerable success in preventing a western spread of the virus in the raccoon population. In 1996, the first year of the incursion of raccoon rabies into Ohio, 13 cases of rabies in raccoons were reported. In 1997, 59 cases of rabies in raccoons were reported. Extensive oral rabies vaccine programs in May and September of 1997 and April 1998 resulted in only 20 raccoons being reported rabid in 1998 (S. Smith, Ohio

Department of Health, personal communication). While the Northeast and the middle Atlantic states, plus Ohio, directed control efforts toward raccoons, the state of Texas was and is still using the bait to target rabies in coyotes and gray foxes. Two rabies epidemics began in that state in 1988, one involving coyotes and dogs in South Texas, the other in gray foxes in Central Texas.[28] In 1995 the Texas Department of Health began a multiyear oral rabies vaccination program in an effort to create a zone of vaccinated coyotes and foxes along the leading edges of the epidemic. Since 1995 through September 1998, more than 8,500,000 doses of Raboral have been distributed by air over 140,000 square miles. Greater than 82% of coyotes tested have shown evidence of an immune response, and canine rabies has declined in South Texas from 166 cases reported in 1994 to 75 in 1996, 15 in 1996, and 3 in 1997. Similar successful results have been noted in the gray fox program: from 188 cases in 1995 to 6 cases in 1997.[28] Through June 1998, only 4 cases of coyote rabies and 12 cases of fox rabies have been reported for the year (G. Fearneyhough, Texas Department of Health, personal communication).

In 1998, the Compendium Committee added Raboral to the list of rabies vaccines licensed for use in the United States. However, the vaccine is restricted for use only in state and federal control programs and is not available to veterinary practitioners.

Captured wild animals that are destined for zoological parks and that are susceptible to rabies should be quarantined for a minimum of 180 days.[17] Although no rabies vaccines are available for such species, many park curators vaccinate some species of animals to protect them from endemic rabies in the surrounding areas. From a biological viewpoint, the vaccines are probably effective in preventing rabies in most mammalian species if administered correctly. However, should such a vaccinated animal be exposed to rabies or if it bites or otherwise exposes a

There are no licensed parenteral rabies vaccines approved for use in wild or zoo-kept wild animals.

41

person under conditions suspicious for rabies, it must be considered as an unvaccinated animal and managed accordingly.

SUMMARY

Timely and effective PrEP will prevent the highly fatal disease of rabies from occurring in most humans and domestic animals, as well as in some species of wild animals that become exposed to the virus. Parenteral rabies vaccines licensed for use in the United States for human and animal use have been shown to be highly safe and effective in numerous controlled clinical trials, as well as from epidemiologic evidence. Specific guidelines from the ACIP are available for rabies vaccine usage for PrEP for humans and should be strictly adhered to for successful prevention of the disease in individuals at risk for exposure.[6] Recommendations from the NASPHV for rabies vaccination of domestic animals are published annually.[17] These animal rabies vaccination guidelines, along with manufacturers' package inserts, should be followed as closely as possible, recognizing that some states or local governments accept different time intervals for revaccinating dogs, cats, and ferrets. Genetically engineered recombinant vaccines are available to governmental agencies for control of the disease in raccoons, foxes, and coyotes. Although rabies is a fatal disease of warm-blooded animals, including humans, the disease can and should be prevented by proper use of the safe and effective vaccines available to the medical professions.

REFERENCES

1. Schneider LG: Spread of virus from the central nervous system, in Baer GM (ed): *The Natural History of Rabies*, ed 2. Boca Raton, CRC Press, 1991, pp 133–144.
2. Fakadu M: Latency and abortive rabies, in Baer GM (ed): *The Natural History of Rabies*, ed 2. Boca Raton, CRC Press, 1991, pp 191–198.
3. World Survey of Rabies No. 32 for the Year 1996, *Rabnet*. WHO/EMC/ZDI/98.4. Geneva, World Health Organization, 1996.
4. Krebs JW, Smith JS, Rupprecht CE, Childs JE: Rabies surveillance in the United States during 1996. *JAVMA* 211(12):1525–1539, 1997.
5. WHO Expert Committee on Rabies, Eighth Report. *WHO Technical Rpt Series 844*. Geneva, World Health Organization, 1992, pp 21–22.
6. Centers for Disease Control and Prevention: Human rabies prevention—United States, 1999. Recommendations of the Advisory Committee on Immunization Practices (ACIP). *MMWR Morb Mortal Wkly Rpt* 48(RR-1):1–21, 1999.
7. Fishbein DB: Rabies in humans, in Baer GM (ed): *The Natural History of Rabies*, ed 2. Boca Raton, CRC Press, 1991, pp 519–549.
8. Hanlon CA, Rupprecht CE: The reemergence of rabies, in Scheld WM, Armstrong D, Hughes JM (eds): *Emerging Infections*. Washington, DC, ASM Press, 1998, pp 59–80.
9. Dreesen DW, Brown J, Sumner JW, Kemp DT: Intradermal use of human diploid cell vaccine for pre-exposure rabies vaccination of humans. *JAVMA* 181(11):1519–1523, 1982.
10. Fishbein DB, Pacer RE, Holmes DF, et al: Rabies preexposure prophylaxis with human diploid cell vaccine: A dose response study. *J Infect Dis* 156(1):50–55, 1987.
11. Bernard KW, Roberts MA, Sumner J, et al: Human diploid cell vaccine. Effectiveness of immunizations with small intradermal doses. *JAMA* 247:1138–1142, 1982.
12. Dreesen DW, Fishbein DB, Kemp DT, Brown J: Two-year comparative trial on the immunogenicity and adverse effects of purified chick embryo cell rabies vaccine for pre-exposure immunizations. *Vaccine* 7:397–400, 1989.
13. Centers for Disease Control. Field evaluations of pre-exposure use of human diploid cell rabies vaccine. *MMWR Morb Mortal Wkly Rpt* 32(46):601–603, 1983.
14. Briggs DJ, Schwenke JR: Longevity of rabies antibody titre in recipients of human diploid cell vaccine. *Vaccine* 10:125–129, 1992.
15. Warrington RJ, Martens CJ, Rubin M, et al: Immunologic studies in subjects with a serum sickness-like illness after immunization with human diploid cell vaccine. *J Allergy Clin Immunol*, pp 605–610, April, 1987.
16. Dreesen DW, Bernard KW, Parker RA, et al: Immune complex-like disease in 23 persons following a booster dose of rabies human diploid cell vaccine. *Vaccine* 4:45–49, 1986.
17. Compendium of Animal Rabies Control, 1999. Report of the National Association of State Public Health Veterinarians Committee. *JAVMA* 214(2):198–202, 1999.
18. Compendium of Animal Rabies Control, 1998. Report of the National Association of State Public Health Veterinarians Committee. *JAVMA* 212(2):213–217, 1998.
19. Eng TR, Fishbein DB: Epidemiologic factors, clinical findings, and vaccination status of rabies in cats and dogs in the United States in 1988. *JAVMA* 197(5):875–878,1990.
20. Petronek GJ: Free-roaming and feral cats—their impact on wildlife and human beings. *JAVMA* 212(2):218–226, 1998.
21. Niezgoda M, Briggs DJ, Shaddock JH, et al: Pathogenesis of experimentally induced rabies in

From a biological viewpoint, vaccines are probably effective in preventing rabies in most mammalian species if administered correctly.

the domestic ferret. *Am J Vet Res* 58(11):1327–1331, 1997.

22. U.S. Government Printing Office: Code of Federal Regulations, Title 9, Part 113, Section 209. Washington, DC, US Government Printing Office, 1998.

23. Greene CE, Dreesen DW: Rabies, in Greene CE (ed): *Infectious Diseases of the Dog and Cat,* ed 2. Philadelphia, WB Saunders, 1998, pp 114–126.

24. Dubielzig RR, Hawkins KL, Miller PE: Myofibroplastic sarcoma organizing at the site of rabies vaccination in the cat. *J Vet Diagn Invest* 5:637–638, 1993.

25. Kass PH, Spangler WL: Epidemiologic evidence for a causal relation between vaccination and fibrosarcoma tumorigenesis in cats. *JAVMA* 203:396–405, 1993.

26. Dreesen DW: Equine rabies. Veterinary Reports. [Solvay Animal Health] 3(2):1–4, 1990.

27. Kieny MP, Lathe R, Drillien R, et al: Expression of the rabies virus glycoprotein from a recombinant vaccinia virus. *Nature* 312:163–166, 1984.

28. Fearneyhough MG: Summary of the Texas oral rabies vaccination program (ORVP). Kingston, Ontario, Canada, Eighth Annual Rabies in the Americas Conference. Nov. 2–6, 1997.

Rabies Postexposure Prophylaxis: Human and Domestic Animal Considerations

Gayne Fearneyhough, BS, DVM
Director, Oral Vaccination Program
Texas Department of Public Health
Austin, Texas

Worldwide, an estimated 40,000 to 100,000 human deaths result from rabies each year.

SINCE THE MIDDLE OF THIS CENTURY, AN AVERAGE OF ONE OR TWO HUMAN RABIES CASES HAVE BEEN REPORTED ANNUALLY IN THE UNITED STATES. HOWEVER, THE 1996 ESTIMATED COST FOR RABIES BIOLOGICALS REQUIRED FOR POSTEXPOSURE PROPHYLAXIS (PEP) FOR PEOPLE EXPOSED TO A RABID OR POTENTIALLY RABID ANIMAL WAS BETWEEN $26.5 MILLION AND $65.3 MILLION.[1] IN THREE STUDIES CONDUCTED SINCE 1980, THE TOTAL ANNUAL EXPENDITURE TO PREVENT RABIES IN THE UNITED STATES WAS FOUND TO BE AT LEAST $230 MILLION AND MAY BE AS MUCH AS $1 BILLION ANNUALLY.[2] A CURSORY ANALYSIS OF THE PUBLIC HEALTH SIGNIFICANCE OF RABIES IN THE UNITED STATES COULD EASILY RESULT IN THE CONCLUSION THAT A DISPROPORTIONATE NUMBER OF RESOURCES ARE ALLOCATED TO THE DISEASE, ESPECIALLY WHEN CASES OF HUMAN RABIES AND RABIES IN DOMESTIC ANIMALS HAVE DECLINED OVER THE LAST 50 YEARS. HOWEVER, A MORE DETAILED EXAMINATION OF THE EPIDEMIOLOGY OF RABIES REVEALS A VALID CAUSE FOR CONCERN, WITH RAPIDLY EXPANDING EPIZOOTICS OF WILDLIFE RABIES IN RACCOONS IN THE EASTERN UNITED STATES, IN FOXES IN TEXAS AND THE NORTHEASTERN UNITED STATES, AND COYOTES IN TEXAS. AN ADDITIONAL CAUSE FOR CONCERN IS THE IDENTIFICATION OF A VIRAL VARIANT TRANSMITTED BY BATS THAT MAY REPRESENT AN INCREASED PUBLIC HEALTH THREAT. THAT THREAT HAS CAUSED MODIFICATION TO THE CENTERS FOR DISEASE CONTROL AND PREVENTION (CDC) RECOMMENDATIONS FOR PEP FOR PEOPLE EXPERIENCING A POTENTIAL EXPOSURE TO A BAT.[3]

Although rabies causes only one or two human deaths annually in the United States, it is important to understand that, worldwide, an estimated 40,000 to 100,000 human deaths result from rabies each year.[4] Consequently, as a society we tend to have a strong and sometimes unreasonable fear of exposure to the rabies virus. That fearful response may be attributed in part to the graphic depiction of the disease by the entertainment industry in motion pictures such as *Old Yeller* and *Cujo.* Fear of rabies may stimulate someone with a potential exposure to rabies to seek medical intervention and, thereby, save a human life. Conversely, fear also causes patients to demand treatment when a threat does not exist and may result in the inappropriate use of valuable medical resources. Practicing veterinarians, human medical professionals, or public health workers may find that they are the most informed participants in a risk analysis process following a potential human or animal exposure to rabies. When administered according to recommendations provided by the Advisory Committee on Immunization Practices (ACIP), PEP has been shown to be essentially 100% effective. Given that rabies is universally fatal, it is essential that accurate and timely decisions be made concerning the administration of PEP.

A 1946 report by the Committee on Animal Health of the National Research Council determined that rabies was a preventable disease and proposed that a coordinated effort to achieve that goal be developed under the leadership of the United States Department of Agriculture (USDA) and individual state veterinarians.[5] Control measures that focused on domestic animal vaccination, local animal control programs, public education, and wildlife depopulation were proposed. In 1938 there were 9,412 cases of rabies reported in animals (mostly in domestic species) and 47 human deaths.[4] As late as 1960 the majority of rabies cases were still reported in domestic species.

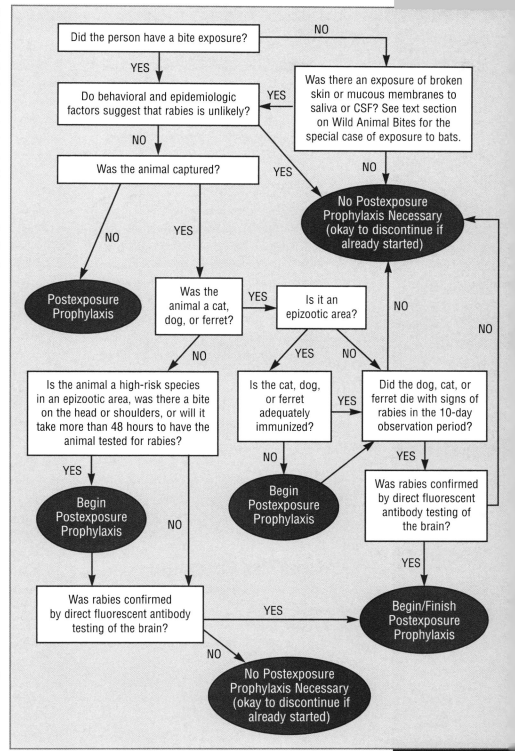

Figure 1—Rabies postexposure prophylaxis decision tree

However, beginning in 1990 there was a dramatic increase in reported cases of wildlife rabies, principally attributed to the raccoon rabies epizootic in the eastern United States. From 1990 to 1993, a 225% increase was reported in raccoon rabies cases (from 1,812 to 5,885) in the mid-Atlantic and northeastern states. By 1996 greater than 90% of the 7,124 animal rabies cases reported in the United States to the CDC were in wildlife species.[1,6]

Although a coordinated national program did not develop, some or all of the principles for rabies control that were proposed in 1946 were employed at the state and local level. It is reasonable to assume that those measures had a favorable impact on the reduction of human and domestic animal rabies cases over the last 50 years. However, the changing face of rabies with the identification of new animal reservoirs and new viral variants has necessitated that rabies control and PEP recommendations constantly evolve. That evolutionary process should employ the application of new technology to continue to prevent human deaths through the appropriate application of PEP and the development of innovative programs to reduce the presence of rabies in wildlife.

RABIES RISK ASSESSMENT

The evaluation process to ascertain an individual's risk of exposure to rabies first involves the determination of whether a bite or nonbite exposure may have occurred. If an exposure has occurred that could result in rabies virus transmission, it is critical that proper wound management techniques be used immediately. The simple process of proper wound cleansing and irrigation with adequate soap and water can reduce the potential for rabies.[7] Assessment of the wound and appropriate use of antibiotic therapy and tetanus prophylaxis should also be considered.

The end result of what can be a complicated risk assessment process is the decision of whether to initiate PEP. A decision to withhold PEP while awaiting the outcome of a laboratory test or the outcome of a quarantine period for the biting domestic animal constitutes a decision to not treat the patient at that time. If a patient has been exposed to rabies, the greatest chance for survival may depend on prompt initiation of PEP. The process of reaching a risk assessment decision can be complicated and clouded by emotional and legal considerations. The following summary of risk assessment considerations is taken from the recommendations of the ACIP and the National Association of State Public Health Veterinarians (NASPHV), as published in the *Compendium of Animal Rabies Control, 1998.*[7,8] These recommendations constitute the minimum criteria that should be considered in evaluating a patient's risk for rabies exposure. Refer to Figure 1 for a rabies PEP decision tree.

Type of Exposure

The principal mechanism of rabies transmission involves a bite wound, which allows the passage of virus-containing saliva across a previously intact skin barrier. Bites to the face and hands carry the highest risk, but the site of the bite should not influence the decision to begin PEP. Nonbite exposure by scratches, abrasions, open wounds, and mucous membranes that are exposed to saliva or other infective material (i.e., brain tissue, cerebrospinal fluid [CSF]) may also constitute an exposure. Petting a rabid animal; exposure of intact skin with blood, urine, or feces of a rabid animal; or contact with fluids that may have been infective but have dried does not constitute an exposure. Nonbite exposure from aerosolized rabies virus in caves, laboratory settings, or organ transplants (i.e., corneas) has occurred but represents very unlikely exposure situations.

The Exposing Animal
Wild Animal Bites

Bites by wild carnivores and bats should

be considered an exposure to rabies and requires initiation of PEP for the patient. The biting animal should be humanely killed immediately and the brain tested for rabies, especially in species that may be defined as high risk for rabies exposure, such as raccoons, skunks, foxes, and bats. The recent epizootic of canine rabies in coyotes along the Texas-Mexico border and the practice of translocating coyotes for hunting purposes may make it prudent to also consider them a high-risk species. PEP may be delayed if the bite occurs in a geographic area of the United States that is free of terrestrial rabies and if the results of immunofluorescence testing will be available within 48 hours. If treatment is initiated and the biting animal is shown not to be rabid, treatment may be discontinued. Exotic animals and valuable specimens that have been confined and have been determined by public health authorities to represent a very limited risk may be quarantined for 30 days in lieu of testing. Rodent and lagomorph species are almost never found to be infected with rabies, and local health departments should be consulted concerning bites by those animal groups. However, rabies in groundhogs accounted for 70% of the 179 cases among rodents reported to the CDC from 1971 through 1988.[7] An analysis of data reported by Krebs and associates during 1991 through 1996 indicates an annual average of 52 cases of rabies in groundhogs, with most of those cases attributed to the raccoon variant of the rabies virus.[9] The Conference of State and Territorial Epidemiologists (CSTE) and the NASPHV consider exotic pets and domestic animals crossbred with wild animals to be wild animals.[8] A bite by any of those animals should be handled as an exposure to a wild animal.

Modifications to PEP recommendations were presented to the ACIP in 1996 because data indicated that bats were associated with an increasing number of human rabies cases. From 1990 through 1996 bat rabies variants were associated with 15 of 17 indigenously acquired cases of human rabies. An identifiable bite was reported in only one of those cases, suggesting that minimal or unnoticed physical contact with bats may result in viral transmission.[1] In situations in which a bat is physically present and the person(s) cannot reasonably exclude the possibility of a bite exposure, PEP should be given unless prompt capture and testing of the bat have excluded rabies virus infection.[10] This recommendation has particular significance for children, mentally challenged adults, and intoxicated individuals who may be unable to responsibly assess whether contact with a bat has occurred. If a bat is found in a room with an unattended child or is found present in a room in which a child or adult was sleeping and physical contact cannot be excluded, PEP should be initiated immediately and, if available, the bat should be tested for rabies. Negative immunofluorescence antibody testing results from a certified laboratory are justification for discontinuing PEP.

Domestic Animal Bites

The NASPHV makes recommendations to be used in the management of animals that bite humans.[8] They can be found on page 83.

Circumstances of the Bite

An unprovoked bite by a domestic animal may constitute an increased risk for rabies in the biting animal and contributes to a decision to initiate PEP for the patient. People fear being bitten by an animal, so it is reasonable to assume that most bites inflicted on humans by domestic animals are not intentionally provoked. However, it is important to emphasize that the human definition of provocation may not be consistent with conditions that elicit aggressive or defensive behavior in a domestic species. Although not often seen as provocative behavior by people, actions such as invading the ill-defined physical territory of an animal, disturbing an animal during eating, staring into the eyes of a dominant animal, playing

Recent data suggest that minimal or unnoticed physical contact with bats may result in viral transmission.

by children that may attempt to force an animal to the ground, or blowing into the face of an animal are but a few examples of human behavior that may produce an aggressive response in a normal animal.

Vaccination Status of the Exposing Animal

Knowledge that a biting domestic animal is currently vaccinated with a vaccine licensed for that species does not remove all concern for involvement of rabies because no vaccine can be considered to be 100% effective. However, animal vaccines licensed for use in the United States have achieved a high level of immunogenicity, and their use in domestic species for which a license has been approved markedly reduces the potential for rabies involvement. Knowledge of a current vaccination in the biting animal, when combined with a lack of epidemiologic evidence of terrestrial rabies in the geographic area and reduced risk associated with conditions of the bite, may allow for justification of a 10-day quarantine period for a biting animal. Utilizing a 10-day quarantine period has obvious benefits to the owner of a valuable animal over euthanizing the animal and testing the brain. If the animal is available for quarantine and the risk assessment process indicates a low probability for rabies, PEP can be delayed for the patient. However, PEP should be initiated immediately at the first sign of rabies in the quarantined animal (Table 1).

RABIES IMMUNIZING PRODUCTS FOR USE IN HUMANS

There are two types of immunizing products for use in humans: (1) immune globulins that provide rapid passive immune protection for a short time (half-life of about 21 days) and (2) vaccines that induce an active immune response, which requires about 7 to 10 days to develop, but immunity may persist for at least 1 year or more. Both types of products should be used concurrently for rabies PEP in those persons who have never received prior immunization against rabies. It is recommended that the package insert be consulted before any of these products are used.[11]

Rabies Immune Globulin

Human rabies immune globulin (HRIG): HRIG (Imogam® Rabies–HT [Pasteur Mérieux Connaught] and BayRab® [Bayer Laboratories]) are antirabies gamma globulin concentrated by cold ethanol fractionation from the plasma of immunized human donors. Rabies neutralizing antibody content is standardized to contain 150 IU/ml. It is supplied in 2 ml (300 IU) and 10 ml (1,500 IU) vials for pediatric and adult use, respectively (Table 2). Imogam Rabies–HT has received an additional heat treatment (HT) step to further reduce the risk of the transmission of known or unknown blood-borne viruses.

Vaccines
Human Diploid Cell Vaccine

Human diploid cell vaccine (HDCV) is an inactivated virus vaccine prepared from rabies virus grown in human diploid cell culture and then inactivated (Table 3). Vaccine is supplied as 1-ml single-dose vials of freeze-dried vaccine with accompanying diluent for intramuscular (IM) injection (Imovax® Rabies Vaccine [Pasteur Mérieux Connaught]) and 0.1-ml single-dose syringes of freeze-dried vaccine with accompanying diluent for preexposure intradermal (ID) use (Imovax® Rabies I.D. [Pasteur Mérieux Connaught]). Both formulations must be used immediately after reconstitution.

Purified Chick Embryo Cell Culture

Purified chick embryo cell (PCEC) culture is a sterile, freeze-dried vaccine obtained by growing the Flury-fixed virus strain, low-egg passage in primary cultures of chicken fibroblasts (Table 3). Purified chick embryo cell culture (RabAvert®,

TABLE 1
Current ACIP Rabies Postexposure Human Prophylaxis Guide[7]

Animal Type	Evaluation and Disposition of Animal	Postexposure Prophylaxis Recommendations
Dogs and cats	Healthy and available for 10 days	Should not begin PEP unless animal develops clinical signs of rabies[a]
	Rabid or suspect rabid	Immediate PEP
	Unknown or escaped	Consult public health officials
Skunks, raccoons, bats, foxes, and most other carnivores; groundhogs	Regarded as rabid unless geographic area is known to be free of rabies or until animal is proved negative by laboratory test[b]	Immediate PEP
Livestock, rodents, and lagomorphs (rabbits and hares)	Consider individually	Consult public health officials
		Bites of squirrels, hamsters, guinea pigs, gerbils, chipmunks, rats, mice, other rodents, rabbits, and hares almost never require antirabies treatment

[a]During the 10-day holding period, begin treatment with HRIG and HDCV or PCEC at first sign of rabies in a dog or cat that has bitten someone. The animal with clinical signs should be euthanized immediately and tested.
[b]The animal should be euthanized and tested as soon as possible. Holding for observation is not recommended. Discontinue vaccine if immunofluorescence test results of the animal are negative.

TABLE 2
Postexposure Treatment Products—Human Rabies Immune Globulin (HRIG)[a]

Product Name	Manufacturer
Imogam®	Pasteur Mérieux Connaught Laboratories
BayRab®	Bayer Laboratories

[a]Administered at time of first dose of vaccine only. Patient weight is needed to determine HRIG dosage. Dosage is 20 IU/kg (2 ml/33 lb).

Chiron Behring GmhH & Co.) is licensed in the United States for IM use in both pre-exposure immunization and PEP. The schedules and dosage for PCEC are the same as for HDCV. It may be used as a booster dose even if another rabies vaccine was used for the primary series.

Serious adverse reactions associated with some rabies vaccines include systemic, anaphylactic, and neuroparalytic reactions. Serious adverse reactions occur at lower rates with HDCV or PCEC vaccines than with previously available types of rabies vaccine.

PEP IMMUNIZATION PROTOCOL

Postexposure antirabies immunization should include administration of both rabies antibody (HRIG) and vaccine (HDCV or PCEC). An exception to this guideline is made for exposed persons who have been previously immunized with the recommended preexposure or postexposure regimens of HDCV or PCEC (or who have been immunized with other types of vaccines and have documented an adequate rabies antibody titer). In those cases, HRIG would not be given and only two doses of vaccine would be given on day 0 and day 3 (Table 4).

The combination of immune globulin and vaccine is recommended for persons not previously immunized for both bite exposures and nonbite exposures, regardless of the interval between exposure and treatment. The sooner treatment is begun after exposure, the better the chance of effectiveness. However, if there was a delay in recognizing a rabies exposure, treatment may be started even months after that exposure occurred.

Five 1.0-ml doses of HDCV or PCEC

Knowledge that a biting domestic animal is currently vaccinated with a vaccine licensed for that species does not remove all concern for involvement of rabies.

TABLE 3
Postexposure Treatment Products—Human Rabies Vaccines

Product Name	Manufacturer
Imovax®—human diploid cell vaccine (HDCV)	Pasteur Mérieux Connaught Laboratories
RabAvert®—purified chick embryo cell (PCEC)	Chiron Behring GmhH & Co.

should be given IM in the deltoid region in adults or on the anterolateral thigh in infants. The ID route should not be used for PEP. The first dose should be given as soon as possible after exposure; additional doses should be given on days 3, 7, 14, and 28 after the first dose. Antibody response following the recommended vaccination regimen has been uniformly satisfactory; therefore, routine postvaccination serologic testing is not normally recommended. However, in unusual instances, such as when the patient is immunodeficient or immunosuppressed, serologic testing (rapid fluorescent focus inhibition test, or RFFIT) is indicated. The RFFIT is available with fast turnaround through the Department of Veterinary Diagnosis, Veterinary Medical Center, Kansas State University, Manhattan, Kansas 66506, telephone: 785-532-5650.

The selection of sites for IM injections of vaccine appears to be critical for vaccine efficacy. In adults and larger children, HDCV or PCEC should be given in the deltoid area. In infants and small children, the anterolateral thigh should be used. In the two laboratory-confirmed cases of human rabies following postexposure treatment with HDCV and HRIG within 24 hours, the HDCV was administered in the gluteal area. Presumably, subcutaneous fat in the gluteal area may interfere with proper IM administration of the vaccine and therefore reduces the immunogenicity of the vaccine.

HRIG is administered only once at the beginning of antirabies prophylaxis to provide immediate antibodies until the patient responds to vaccination with active production of antibodies. If HRIG was not given at the initiation of vaccination, it can be given up to the eighth day after the first dose of vaccine. From the eighth day on, HRIG is not indicated because an antibody response to the vaccine is presumed to have occurred.

The recommended dose of HRIG is 20 IU/kg or approximately 9 IU/lb (2 ml/33 lb) of body weight. As much of the full dose of HRIG as possible should be thoroughly infiltrated into and around the wound(s). Any remaining volume should be administered IM at a site distant from vaccine inoculation. No more than the recommended dose of HRIG should be given because it may partially suppress active production of antibody.

PEP TREATMENT OUTSIDE THE UNITED STATES

If PEP treatment is begun outside the United States with locally produced biologicals, it may be desirable to provide additional treatment when the patient reaches the United States. For specific advice in such cases, contact the local health department.

POSTEXPOSURE THERAPY OF PREVIOUSLY IMMUNIZED PERSONS

Preexposure immunization does not remove the need for PEP; it merely reduces the extent of treatment. Upon exposure to rabies, an immunized person who was vaccinated with the recommended regimen of HDCV or PCEC or who has previously demonstrated rabies antibody should receive two IM doses (1.0 ml each) of HDCV or PCEC, one immediately and one 3 days later (Table 4). HRIG should not be given in these cases. Full primary postexposure antirabies treatment (HRIG plus five doses of HDCV or PCEC) may be necessary in the case of unknown immune status in a previously vaccinated person who did not receive the recommended HDCV or PCEC regimen. In such cases, if antibody can be

TABLE 4
Rabies Postexposure Prophylaxis Schedule, United States[11]

Patient Vaccination Status	Treatment	Regimen[a]
Not previously vaccinated	Local wound cleansing	All postexposure treatment should begin with immediate, thorough cleansing of all wounds with soap and water.
	HRIG	20 IU/kg body weight. As much as possible of the full dose should be infiltrated into and around the wound(s), and the remainder should be administered IM at an anatomic site distant from vaccine administration. HRIG should not be administered in the same syringe as vaccine. Because HRIG may partially suppress active production of antibody, no more than the recommended dose should be given.
	Vaccine	HDCV or PCEC 1.0 ml IM (deltoid area[b]) on days 0, 3, 7, 14, and 28.
Previously vaccinated[c]	Local wound cleansing	All postexposure treatment should begin with immediate thorough cleansing of all wounds with soap and water.
	HRIG	HRIG should not be administered.
	Vaccine	HDCV or PCEC 1.0 ml IM (deltoid area[b]) on days 0 and 3.

[a]These regimens are applicable for all age groups, including children.
[b]The deltoid area is the only acceptable site of vaccination for adults and older children. For younger children, the outer aspect of the thigh may be used. Vaccine should never be administered in the gluteal area.
[c]Any person with a history of preexposure vaccination with HDCV or PCEC, prior postexposure prophylaxis with HDCV or PCEC, or previous vaccination with any other type of rabies vaccine and documented history of antibody response to the prior vaccination.

demonstrated in a serum sample collected before vaccine is given, treatment can be discontinued after at least two doses of HDCV or PCEC.

ACCIDENTAL HUMAN EXPOSURE TO ANIMAL RABIES VACCINE

Accidental inoculation or vaccine contact with mucous membranes may occur to individuals during administration of rabies vaccines to animals. Such exposure to inactivated rabies vaccine constitutes no known rabies hazard.

PRECAUTIONS AND CONTRAINDICATIONS
Immunosuppression

Corticosteroids and other immunosuppressive agents, antimalarials, and immunosuppressive illnesses (such as HIV infection) can interfere with the development of active immunity and predispose the patient to the development of rabies. Immunosuppressive agents should not be administered during postexposure therapy, unless essential for the treatment of other conditions. When rabies PEP is administered to persons receiving corticosteroids or other immunosuppressive therapy or to persons having an immunosuppressive illness, it is especially important that the patient be tested for rabies antibody to ensure that an adequate response has developed.

Pregnancy

Because of the potential consequences of an inadequately treated rabies exposure and limited data indicating that fetal abnormalities have been associated with rabies vaccination, pregnancy is not considered a con-

The selection of sites for IM injections of vaccine appears to be critical for vaccine efficacy.

traindication to PEP. If a substantial unavoidable risk of exposure to rabies exists, preexposure prophylaxis may also be indicated during pregnancy.

Allergies

Persons with histories of hypersensitivity should be given rabies vaccines with caution. When a patient with a history suggesting hypersensitivity to HDCV or PCEC must be given that vaccine, antihistamines can be given; epinephrine should be readily available to counteract anaphylactic reactions, and the person should be carefully observed.

MANAGEMENT OF PETS EXPOSED TO RABID ANIMALS

The management of cases of domestic animals exposed to rabies can be difficult because of the lack of an immediate perceived threat to human life. The exposure incident obviously could later result in a human exposure if the domestic animal should develop rabies. Therefore, the recommendation normally has been to sacrifice the exposed animal. Management of these cases may also be further complicated by emotional value of the animal and conflict over the rights of ownership of private property and the disposition of that property when little or no human health risk exists.

The NASPHV's *Compendium on Animal Rabies Control, 1998,* recommends postexposure management for animals exposed to a rabid animal[8] as indicated on page 82.

Confusion has occurred with respect to (1) the 10-day observation period for a dog, cat, or ferret that has bitten or scratched a human and (2) the period of strict isolation required for an unvaccinated dog, cat, or ferret that has been exposed to a rabid animal. Generally, when clinical symptoms of rabies are first evident, the rabies virus also becomes present in the saliva and a dog, cat, or ferret will survive no more than 3 to 5 days. If the animal is clinically normal 10 days after the biting incident, it is not considered likely for rabies virus to have been present in its saliva at the time of the bite. Therefore, exposure to rabies virus could not have resulted from the bite, and PEP is not indicated. A dog, cat, or ferret may develop rabies more than 10 days after having bitten a person but the animal would not be considered to have been infective at the time of the bite.

The 10-day observation period is not applicable for a dog, cat, or ferret exposed to a rabid animal. The average incubation time for rabies in those species is generally 3 to 8 weeks; therefore, an observation period of 45 days for vaccinated animals and 180 days for unvaccinated animals is recommended. Consequently, the 10-day observation period is useful in ensuring that a dog, cat, or ferret was not able to transmit rabies at the time of a biting incident, but it is not applicable for those species under observation after an exposure to a rabid animal.

PEP JUSTIFICATION FOR DOMESTIC ANIMALS

The primary concern of the risk assessment process to determine the appropriateness of PEP for a human patient must be the patient's safety. Rabies is universally fatal, so there is a tendency to administer PEP to the human patient when there may be even a limited potential for rabies exposure. That conservative approach to management of the human patient has also resulted in recommendations for sacrificing an animal exposed to or potentially exposed to rabies. Such recommendations are not usually based on a callous approach to the value of the animal but rather on a concern that the exposed animal might later develop rabies and represent a serious public health threat. The reluctance to advocate the use of PEP in animals is also complicated by the fact that there is very limited scientific data published to demonstrate the effectiveness of PEP when administered to domestic animals.

A 1996 study by Clark and Wilson does

provide data to demonstrate the effectiveness of PEP in unvaccinated domestic animals.[12] This retrospective study was conducted using two PEP protocols on 1,345 unvaccinated domestic animals that were exposed to rabies and reported to the Texas Department of Health over a 16-year period. The first PEP protocol was used from 1979 through 1987 and involved 713 animals (440 dogs; 57 cats; 145 cattle; 53 horses; and 18 sheep, goats, and pigs). The exposed animals were immediately vaccinated and revaccinated 1 month prior to release from a 6-month period of isolation (there is no USDA-licensed vaccine for goats and pigs). The second protocol was used from 1988 through 1994 and involved 632 animals (406 dogs; 106 cats; 69 cattle; 43 horses; 7 sheep, pigs or goats; and 1 llama). In the second protocol, the exposed animals were vaccinated immediately and given booster vaccinations during the third and eighth weeks of a 90-day isolation period (there is no USDA-licensed vaccine for llamas). This study determined that 711 of 713 animals (99.7%) given PEP using the first protocol and 629 of 632 animals (99.5%) given the second protocol survived.

Another study in 1991 by Blancou and associates to determine the efficacy of the human PEP protocol used 68 sheep experimentally infected with fox rabies virus.[13] The infected sheep were divided into three groups and were given cell culture vaccine on days 0, 3, 7, and 14; HRIG at 26 IU/kg on day 0; or a combination of vaccine and immune globulin. Seventy-one percent of the controls died; the treatment protocol using a combination of vaccine and immune globulin was found to be 100% effective. These results seem to indicate that there may be justification for PEP for domestic animals. Additional studies are needed to identify animal PEP protocols capable of producing a high level of survivability, conforming to public health concerns, and yet being economically applicable to domestic animals.

SUMMARY

The emphasis on rabies control and prevention in the United States seems to be a function of our perception of proximity of the threat. Wildlife rabies epizootics within a state may be of little concern to the uninformed urban dweller. Additionally, many parts of the western United States are free of terrestrial rabies and, were it not for the presence of bat rabies, people in those areas would likely interpret rabies control as a very minor public health concern. It is essential that federal, state, and local public health programs emphasize the importance of rabies control through activities that include rabies education, sponsorship of legislated requirements for domestic animal vaccination, support for local animal control programs, and promotion of recommendations that encourage the appropriate use of PEP. We are almost guaranteed that rabies will remain a major public health issue well into the next century because of expanding wildlife rabies epizootics, identification of new rabies viral variants with increased public health concern, emotional and legal concerns associated with rabies exposure, and increasing national cost associated with rabies control and prevention. However, the development of new laboratory technology that allows an understanding of the epidemiology of the rabies virus based on an evolving genetic history and the interrelationship with wildlife reservoirs will allow access to valuable tools for rabies control. That technology, when combined with programs utilizing new developments in oral rabies vaccine that can immunize whole populations of wildlife reservoirs, offers encouragement in our effort to control one of the diseases of antiquity.[14]

ACKNOWLEDGMENTS

The author would like to thank Dr. Erik Svenkerud and Pamela J. Wilson of the Texas Department of Health for their assistance and editorial comment.

If an animal is clinically normal 10 days after a biting incident, it is not considered possible for rabies virus to have been present in its saliva at the time of the bite.

REFERENCES

1. Krebs JW, Long-Marin SC, Childs JE: Causes, cost, and estimates of rabies postexposure prophylaxis treatment in the United States. *Journal of Public Health Management and Practice* 4(5):56–62, 1998.

2. Fishbein DB, Robinson LE: Rabies. *N Engl J Med* 329(22):1632–1638, 1993.

3. Childs JE, Krebs JW, Rupprecht CE: Epidemiology of bat rabies In the USA. Kingston, Ontario, Canada, Eighth Annual International Meeting of Rabies in the Americas. November 2–6, 1997.

4. Rupprecht CE, Smith JS, Fekadu M, Childs JE: The ascension of wildlife rabies: A cause for public health concern or intervention? *Emerg Infect Dis* October–December 1(4):107–113, 1995.

5. National Research Council: Committee on animal health report: Rabies and its control. *JAVMA* CVIII (830):293–302, 1946.

6. Rupprecht CE, Smith JS, Krebs J, et al: Current issues in rabies prevention in the United States, health dilemmas, public coffers, private interests. *Public Health Rep* 111:400–407, 1996.

7. Centers for Disease Control and Prevention: Rabies prevention—United States, 1991, recommendations of the Immunization Practices Advisory Committee (ACIP). *MMWR Morb Mortal Wkly Rep* 40(RR-3):1–19, 1991.

8. National Association of State Public Health Veterinarians, Inc: Compendium of Animal Rabies Control, 1998. *MMWR Morb Mortal Wkly Rep* 47(RR-9):1–9, May 29, 1998.

9. Krebs J W, Smith JS, Rupprecht CE, Childs JE: Rabies surveillance in the United States during 1996. *JAVMA* 211(12):1525–1539, 1997.

10. Centers for Disease Control and Prevention: Rabies prevention. *MMWR Morb Mortal Wkly Rep* 445:209, 1996.

11. Texas Department of Health: Rabies prevention in Texas 1997. Texas Department of Health Publ, stock no. 6-108,1997.

12. Clark KA, Wilson PJ: Postexposure rabies prophylaxis and preexposure rabies vaccination failure in domestic animals. *JAVMA* 208(11): 1827–1830, 1996.

13. Blancou J, Baltazar RS, Molli I: Effective postposure treatment of rabies-infected sheep with rabies immune globulin and vaccine. *Vaccine* 9(6):432–437, 1991.

14. Fearneyhough MG, Wilson PJ, Clark KA, et al: Results of an oral rabies vaccination program for coyotes. *JAVMA* 212(4):498–502, 1998.

The Diagnosis of Rabies

Charles V. Trimarchi, MS
Director, Rabies Laboratory
New York State Department of Health
Albany, New York

Deborah J. Briggs, PhD
Professor/Director, Rabies Laboratory
Kansas State University College of Veterinary Medicine
Manhattan, Kansas

PROPER MANAGEMENT OF EVERY RABIES-RELATED INCIDENT DERIVES ITS IMPORTANCE FROM THE STATUS OF OUR CONQUEST OF THIS DREAD DISEASE TO DATE: RABIES HAS BECOME A PREVENTABLE INFECTION OF HUMANS AND DOMESTIC ANIMALS BY PREEXPOSURE AND POSTEXPOSURE PROPHYLAXIS, BUT IT REMAINS A FATAL, INCURABLE INFECTION ONCE SYMPTOMS BEGIN. THE VALUE OF A CONFIRMED RABIES DIAGNOSIS IN THE PREVENTION OF RABIES MORTALITY IS OBVIOUS. LESS OBVIOUS, BUT EQUALLY VALUABLE TO RABIES CONTROL, ARE RELIABLE NEGATIVE RESULTS THAT PREVENT UNNECESSARY HUMAN EXPOSURE TO THE RISKS OF VACCINATION, WASTEFUL EXPENDITURE OF SCARCE AND EXPENSIVE BIOLOGICS, AND NEEDLESS EUTHANASIA OR LENGTHY QUARANTINE OF COMPANION ANIMALS. RECENT ADVANCES IN THE DEVELOPMENT OF MORE SENSITIVE PROCEDURES FOR ANTEMORTEM DIAGNOSIS OF RABIES IN HUMANS WILL HELP PREVENT AVOIDABLE EXPOSURES TO HEALTHCARE PERSONNEL. THE ABILITY TO IDENTIFY THE VARIANT OF RABIES VIRUS RESPONSIBLE FOR ANIMAL AND HUMAN RABIES CASES AIDS IN THE DEVELOPMENT OF EXPOSURE DEFINITION GUIDELINES AND THE TARGETING OF RABIES CONTROL PROGRAMS. WHEN THE VETERINARIAN, PHYSICIAN, AND PUBLIC HEALTH PRACTITIONER ARE CALLED UPON TO MANAGE A POSSIBLE HUMAN OR DOMESTIC ANIMAL RABIES CASE OR A POSSIBLE EXPOSURE TO RABIES, IT IS PARAMOUNT THAT THEY USE THE LABORATORY DIAGNOSIS OF THE DISEASE EFFECTIVELY AS A FOUNDATION FOR CRITICAL AND OFTEN DIFFICULT DECISIONS. TO DO SO, THESE HEALTHCARE PROFESSIONALS NEED A CLEAR UNDERSTANDING OF THE CAPABILITIES AND LIMITATIONS OF THE MODERN RABIES LABORATORY.

It is paramount that the veterinarian, physician, and public health practitioner use the laboratory diagnosis of rabies as a foundation for critical and often difficult decisions in managing a possible rabies case or possible exposure to rabies.

ROLES OF RABIES DIAGNOSIS

Postmortem diagnosis of rabies in animals is most commonly performed to identify rabies infection in suspect animals that have bitten or otherwise exposed a human or a domestic animal to the disease. Not all biting animals need to be killed and tested. A dog, cat, or ferret that has bitten a person but is wanted by the owner and is not demonstrating signs of rabies infection can be confined and observed daily for 10 days. If, however, the animal dies or signs of rabies develop during the observation period, it must be immediately euthanized and examined. Similarly, when a 10-day confinement of the offending animal is not possible (if it is symptomatic or has died) or is inappropriate (a wild or exotic species with suspected rabies), the animal must be humanely euthanized and tested.[1] Because the modern rabies laboratory can provide reliable results on the day of receipt of the specimen, the physician's decision to provide or withhold rabies treatment after a bite from a suspect animal can commonly be predicated on the postmortem examination. Alternatively, if a delay in testing for rabies is unavoidable, it may be appropriate to initiate rabies treatment. Subsequently, negative results from a reliable laboratory would justify terminating postexposure treatment.

Wild animals, especially bats, foxes, skunks, and raccoons, that have bitten or otherwise potentially exposed a human should be tested immediately. Rabies exposure is defined as the introduction of rabies virus into a bite wound, into an open cut in the skin, or onto mucous membranes.[1] Rabies virus is generally found in concentrations sufficient for infection only in the saliva, salivary glands, and brains of rabid animals. Therefore, contamination from other organs and body fluids is usually not considered a rabies exposure. Because rabies is a disease affecting mammals, it is never necessary to test arthropods, amphibians, reptiles, or birds. In the United States, small rodents including mice, rats, and squirrels are essentially free of rabies, and therefore routine examination is not required; exceptions include rodents involved in unprovoked attacks in rabies-endemic areas and larger rodents such as woodchucks, muskrats, and beavers.[2]

Diagnosis of rabies in animals provides surveillance information on the distribution and prevalence of rabies in wildlife populations and in domestic animals. These data are used in the development of guidelines for animal bite management when the offending animal is not available for observation or testing. The rabies laboratory supports surveillance programs for the disease in wildlife to aid in the proper allocation, targeting, and evaluation of rabies control programs, such as the efforts to vaccinate wildlife with oral baits. Rabies diagnosis is also performed to aid in the differential diagnosis of encephalitis in domestic animals, even in the absence of human or animal exposure.

The laboratory diagnosis of rabies in humans is an important means of evaluating the etiology of human encephalitis. Despite the dire prognosis in rabies infection, testing should be carried out in all cases of acute, progressive encephalitis, even in the absence of a history of bite exposure.[3] Antemortem diagnosis is a valuable tool to permit early identification and postexposure treatment of family and healthcare staff potentially exposed by contact with the patient's saliva and to prepare family for the invariably fatal outcome of the disease. Postmortem diagnosis of rabies in cases of fatal encephalitis of unknown etiology is critical in gaining greater knowledge of the prevalence of rabies encephalitis in humans, the frequency of failure of preexposure and postexposure vaccination, and the probable vectors and variants that pose the greatest risk to human health.

By using methods that permit the antigenic and genetic characterization of isolates, the rabies laboratory can now identify the rabies virus variants responsible for epizootics as well as for individual cases of rabies in animals and humans. Rabies variant identification yields a greater knowledge of the epizootiologic relationships of virus and vectors, permitting the development of more effective animal contact guidelines and rabies control strategies. Reliable assays to demonstrate and quantify rabies antibody in the serum of humans and animals are performed at many rabies laboratories and serve numerous functions in rabies diagnosis and control.

DIAGNOSIS OF RABIES IN ANIMALS

Rabies is a neurotropic virus that invades the central nervous system (CNS) after a variable and sometimes long incubation period. It produces an acute, progressive encephalitis that culminates in death. Rabies diagnosis can be achieved with 100% sensitivity only by the postmortem examination of brain tissue. Throughout most of the prolonged incubation period of rabies there is no means to diagnose infection—there is no rise in circulating antibody titer, and neither rabies virus, its antigens, nor rabies RNA can be reliably identified because of limited and unpredictable distribution during the retrograde axoplasmal movement of the virus from the site of the exposure to the CNS during rabies pathogenesis (discussed in detail in Dr. Ceccaldi's paper on p. 12). However, modern methods can identify the presence of rabies virus in the brain of a rabid animal that dies or is euthanized during, or up to several days before the onset of, the clinical signs of the disease. Therefore, after an exposure, when a decision is made to sacrifice and test the animal for rabies infection, it is never necessary to delay testing for further development of the disease to achieve a reliable diagnosis. Most importantly, centrifugal spread of the virus from the CNS to the salivary glands (and therefore a potentially infectious bite) does not precede the appearance of demonstrable rabies antigen in the brain.[4] Therefore, a negative result of brain examination by acceptable methods ensures that the bite of the animal could not have caused an exposure to rabies.

Specimen Collection, Preservation, and Submission

The distribution of rabies virus and its antigens in the brain varies with species, nature of the exposure, and variant of rabies virus. However, generally the hippocampi, the cerebellum, and the brain stem constitute the best diagnostic samples, and ideally areas of each section are examined to provide a reliable negative report. Therefore, the intact head constitutes the preferred diagnostic sample for the postmortem diagnosis of rabies in animals. An animal can be euthanized for rabies examination by any humane means, including barbiturate and nonbarbiturate injectables and gases, that does not damage the cranium. Immediately following euthanasia, the specimen should be preserved by refrigeration until it arrives at the laboratory. Should refrigeration not be possible, freezing is an acceptable but less desirable alternative—a single freezing and thawing will not prevent reliable diagnosis, but freezing will make the dissection more difficult and may delay the test. Repeated freeze-thaw cycles can damage the specimen. The head should be removed from the neck before the first vertebra, with caution to avoid contaminated injury or creation of infectious aerosols. Those capturing suspected rabid animals or handling and decapitating the carcass should receive rabies preexposure immunization.[1] For very small animals, such as bats, the entire animal should be submitted to avoid damage to the animal's CNS during decapitation. For large livestock species including cattle and equines, sample portions of the brain stem and cerebellum can be removed through the foramen magnum.[5]

Ideally, the specimen should be directly and immediately transported to the laboratory. Specimens also can be shipped by parcel delivery if properly packaged and labeled. Some states have standardized rabies specimen containers for shipping heads to the laboratory. Otherwise, the specimen must be sealed in two heavy (4 mil) plastic bags, individually sealed by knotting. The double-bagged head should then be placed in another bag, similarly sealed, containing several hard-frozen gel-refrigerant packs. This in turn must be contained in an inner Styrofoam box within a wax-treated outer cardboard box. An envelope attached to the outside of the container should contain a fully completed standard rabies specimen history form, if available. If no form is available, provide all the significant information. Include the names, addresses, and telephone numbers of the owner and complainant. List all humans and animals in contact, as well as information on the clinical observations, date of death or means of euthanasia, exact location of capture, and information on the person or agency to receive the report. Generally, reports of rabies-positive specimens are made immediately by telephone. Reporting practices vary widely, however, and the submitter should ascertain local practice.

Necropsy and Dissection

If the entire head is received for examination, the flesh is removed from the cranium and one anterior and two lateral cuts are made in the cranium by chisel or saw to permit the calvarium to be reflected posteriorly. After removal of the meninges, the left and right horns of the hippocampus, the cerebellum, and the brain stem are removed. An alternative method, useful for surveillance-only examinations, employs the removal of a core of brain tissue by inserting a soda straw or similar hollow tube into the foramen magnum and advancing it forward to capture samples of the brain stem, cerebellum, and hippocampus, which can then be forced out of the straw and used for slide and suspension preparation.[6] Touch impressions or slip smears of each tissue are made on microscope slides immediately. A 10% suspension of a mixture of the diagnostic tissues is also made in suitable diluents for animal inoculation or cell culture virus isolation. A sample of each brain tissue is saved at –70°C for further testing.

Histologic Examination

Following Louis Pasteur's demonstration in the late 1800s that rabies was caused by an agent that can be transmitted by the inoculation of infected CNS tissues, Adolchi Negri reported in 1903 a specific diagnostic brain lesion for rabies infection. These intracytoplasmic, acidophilic inclusion bodies can be demonstrated best in the Purkinje cells of the cerebellum and in the pyramidal cells of the hippocampus[7] of the suspect animal by microscopic examination of tissue stained with basic fuchsin and methylene blue[8] or hematoxylin and eosin.[9] The prevalence and size of Negri bodies are related to the species of animal, variant of rabies virus, and duration of the clinical period before death or euthanasia. Although demonstration of these pathognomonic inclusions is very specific and, coupled with evidence of encephalitic inflammatory response, provides a reliable positive rabies diagnosis when issued by an experienced pathologist, the sensitivity of the method is poor: Numerous histologic surveys indicate that 25% or more of rabid animals have no demonstrable Negri bodies, indicating the severe limitation of this diagnostic method for medical decisions.[7]

Direct Immunofluorescence for Rabies Antigen

The combination of speed with specificity and a sensitivity often approaching 100% makes the fluorescent antibody test (FAT) the standard and preferred procedure for the diagnosis of rabies. After fixation for 1 to 4 hours in acetone at –20°C, microscope slides of brain from the suspect animal are flooded with diagnostic fluorescent reagent. These reagents are made by the conjugation of fluorescein isothiocyanate (FITC) to purified IgG specific for rabies nucleocapsid protein. Historically, the antibodies were extracted from antiserum of rabbit, hamster, or horse origin from a rabies-hyperimmune donor. The development of highly specific and easily, continuously produced mouse monoclonal antibodies has permitted development of highly specific diagnostic reagents employing a cocktail of several of these antibodies. After a 30-minute incubation at 37°C in a moist incubator, the diagnostic reagent is thoroughly washed off in multiple saline baths. FITC-conjugated antibodies remain attached to the brain film only where rabies nucleocapsid protein is present. After air drying, the slides are examined using a light microscope fitted with a mercury vapor or xenon lamp and appropriate excitation and barrier filters to show FITC-labeled structures as yellow-green fluorescent objects against a dark background. Rabies-specific staining in brain tissue appears as characteristic round or oval intracytoplasmic inclusions most prominent in the large neurons of the cerebellum, hippocampus, and brain stem (Figure 1).[10]

The sensitivity of rabies immunofluorescence testing can be comparable or superior to isolation procedures. Important factors in the avoidance of false-negative results in rabies diagnosis include the use of proper scientific controls for all procedures, diagnostic conjugate quality and proper dilution, and lamp and microscope performance. The specificity of the procedure also can approach 100% agreement with virus isolation, providing good quality control is used to avoid cross-contamination, along with proper wash and conjugate-diluent selection to minimize nonspecific fluorescence and the selected application of laboratory tests for immunofluorescence specificity. The diagnosis of rabies in animals is not a Clinical Laboratory Improvement Amendment (CLIA) '88 analyte; therefore, proficiency testing is not mandatory. Nevertheless, voluntary rabies proficiency testing programs were conducted periodically from 1973 to 1992 and each year since 1994. The recent performance of rabies diagnostic laboratories enrolled in proficiency testing in the United States has been excellent when evaluating panels of rabies-positive and -negative test slides by the direct FAT. Consensus has been greatest among participants for strong positive and negative test samples. Discrepancies have occurred mainly with very weakly positive slides.[11] The most important factor for efficacy of the rabies FAT is the laboratory's recruitment and retention of properly trained and experienced microscopists.[12] The measure of the value and reliability of the FAT

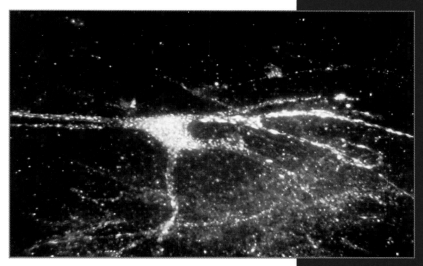

is demonstrated by the absence of any known human rabies cases in the United States when rabies postexposure treatment was withheld based on an immunofluorescence-negative laboratory report.

In practice, the main barrier to sensitive diagnosis by immunofluorescence is a poor-quality sample. Brain tissue exposure to chemical fixative, repeated freeze-thaw cycles, or elevated temperatures can denature or mask the rabies antigens recognized by the diagnostic reagents. Decomposition affects the sensitivity of all rabies diagnostic procedures. Immunofluorescence tests may remain positive for a period after isolation of virus is no longer possible.[13] Evidence of rabies infection by FAT on decomposed or mutilated tissue fragments supports a valid rabies-positive report. One of the most difficult diagnostic decisions is that of determining at what stage of decomposition it is no longer possible to issue a reliable negative rabies report. Certainly, once the CNS has become foul-smelling, green, and partially liquefied, negative results are invalid. Although the rabies FAT can be applied to demonstrate rabies antigen in a wide variety of tissues, mutilation of the specimen by trauma to the extent that the necessary sample regions of cerebellum, brain stem, and hippocampus are not available or are unrecognizable also precludes a reliable negative result. Generally, it is not possible for labo-

Figure 1—Rabies virus antigen in intracytoplasmic inclusions in cell body and dendrites of a large neuron of the brain stem of a horse. (Direct immunofluorescent staining, ×160.)

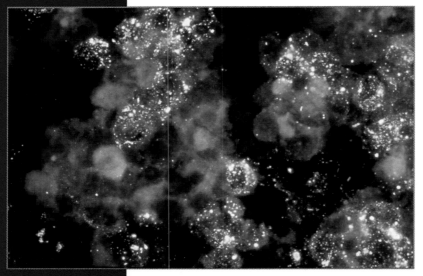

Figure 2—
Rabies-infected
neuroblastoma
cell sheet of tissue
culture virus
isolation test.
(Direct
immunofluorescent
staining with
Evans blue
counterstain,
×320.)

ratory personnel, based solely on a verbal description, to determine before the dissection whether a decomposed or mutilated specimen may be testable. Therefore, for important specimens, unless it is clear that the carcass is in the last stages of decomposition or is mutilated to the extent that no recognizable CNS exists, it is wise to submit compromised specimens to the laboratory for evaluation of suitability.

Virus Isolation

Despite the proven sensitivity and reliability of the FAT for rabies diagnosis, the dire consequences of false-negative results in cases of human exposure support a continued practice of using rabies virus isolation as a backup, confirmatory procedure. It may be used as a general quality-control procedure or applied only to instances of bites to humans from highly suspect animals. In either case it serves to sustain confidence in the reliability of the FAT results and to exonerate the microscopist from the full burden of responsibility. Virus isolation and propagation are also critical components for identification of viral variants and production of diagnostic reagents. In vitro and in vivo methods are both widely used.

The mouse inoculation test (MIT), introduced for diagnostic purposes in 1935, is a very sensitive and reproducible procedure.

Portions of the same tissues that are used for the microscopic examination are ground into a suspension employing a diluent of physiologic salt solution containing serum and antibiotic supplements. The suspension is inoculated intracerebrally into neonatal or weanling Swiss albino mice. The mice are carefully observed daily for 30 days for evidence of rabies infection. Mice developing illness during the observation period are immediately euthanized, and the brains are examined by FAT. The value of the MIT is its ability to detect small quantities of rabies virus in even very weakly positive specimens.[13] It is also applicable to mutilated and decomposed samples. Its weakness lies in the common 7- to 18-day period between inoculation and recognized illness in the mice—if treatment were withheld after a bite because of a false-negative FAT, detection by this backup method would occur after a period that would cause great concern about vaccine failure.[14]

The delayed results of the MIT can be avoided in the modern diagnostic laboratory by the isolation and identification of rabies virus on continuous cell culture. The brain tissue from the suspect animal is ground into a suspension in a cell culture medium as diluent. The suspension is incubated for 1 to several days after inoculation onto a monolayer of cells of a continuous cell line selected for its susceptibility to infection with rabies virus, generally a mouse neuroblastoma cell culture. The cell monolayers are then washed, fixed in cold acetone or a formalin-methanol mix, and then examined by FAT (Figure 2). If infectious rabies virus is present in the brain tissue, characteristic intracytoplasmic inclusions of rabies antigen will be observed in fluorescent foci in the cells. The sensitivity of the procedure is comparable to that of the FAT and the MIT.[15] Because results are available within a few days of receipt of the specimen, it serves as a much better means of confirming negative FAT results, as a false-negative FAT would be recognized in a period of time permitting treatment initiation without concern of vaccination failure.

Other Methods of Antigen Detection

When the CNS has been exposed to formalin or other fixatives, standard FAT and virus isolation procedures are not applicable. Advances have recently increased the sensitivity of direct and indirect immunofluorescence and immunohistochemical procedures applied to fixed tissue. Digestion of the tissue with enzymes such as proteinase prior to staining can expose antigenic sites formerly masked by bonds resulting from fixation.[16] Use of avidin-biotin complex amplification and high-affinity monoclonal antibodies for the first label have improved the performance of these procedures such that they may be approaching the reliability of FAT (Figure 3).[17] Further evaluation is necessary before negative results on chemically fixed tissues can be used for public health decisions. When applicable, confirmatory testing of fixed tissues by another sensitive technique, such as reverse transcription polymerase chain reaction (RT-PCR), is appropriate.

Enzyme-linked immunosorbent assays (ELISA) have been developed for the rapid and simple diagnosis of viral infections. Such a system exists for rabies detection, and the most recent methods (avidin-biotin amplified) show promise of improved sensitivity, approaching that of FAT and virus-isolation.[18] They offer the advantages of automated reading and good reliability on partially decomposed tissues, offering field condition applicability. Although these techniques can be used as a backup to FAT examination and for epizootiologic surveillance testing, they are not widely used in U.S. public health laboratories.

Molecular Methods

The most direct methods for the molecular diagnosis of rabies employ probes for the presence of existing rabies virus RNA in

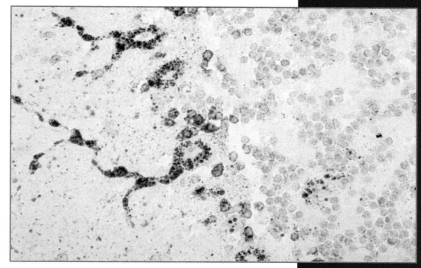

tissue samples. These methods, using dot or blot hybridization assays, generally lack sufficient sensitivity to show the presence of rabies RNA among the total RNAs of the sample, except in the more heavily infected samples.[19]

A more sensitive and useful technique is the RT-PCR. RNA extracted directly from infected brain material is reversely transcribed to complementary DNA (cDNA), which is then amplified by PCR. RT-PCR requires primers, short synthesized oligonucleotide sequences derived from conserved regions of the rabies genome, usually from the nucleoprotein, or N protein, gene. The most sensitive type of PCR is a nested PCR in which a second round of amplification is performed on the initial PCR product using primers internal to the original primers.[20] The products of PCR amplification of the rabies genome can be detected and analyzed in numerous ways. The product can be visualized directly in agarose gels stained with ethidium bromide following electrophoresis, or it can be indirectly detected by using DNA probes revealed by radioactive labels, digoxigenin immunologic detection, or enzymatic revelation with indicators such as alkaline phosphatase.

Molecular diagnosis has important applications (1) in the antemortem diagnosis of human rabies,[21] (2) when paired with re-

Figure 3—Avidin-biotin–amplified immunoperoxidase staining of rabies virus antigen in a frozen section of cerebellum. Note the labeled intracytoplasmic inclusions throughout the flask-shaped Purkinje cells and their dendrites (×160).

Antemortem rabies

diagnosis should

be attempted in

all cases of acute,

progressive human

encephalitis of

unknown etiology.

striction fragment length polymorphism (RFLP) or with nucleotide sequencing analysis in the epizootiologic investigations of rabies,[22] (3) as a sensitive backup test to FAT. However, its current use in routine rabies diagnosis is limited. For a number of reasons, the FAT is unlikely to be replaced by RT-PCR. The FAT test for rabies antigen in brain tissue is rapid, sensitive, specific, easily performed, and relatively inexpensive. In the United States, no human case of rabies has ever been attributed to contact with an animal found negative for rabies by FAT on brain material. Tests for sensitivity and specificity of FAT by comparison to virus isolation approach 100%.[23] Although nested PCR can be 100 to 1,000 times more sensitive than FAT, this extreme sensitivity brings with it a need for extraordinary quality control practices to avoid false-positive results. Small fragments of RNA generated by tissue processing during necropsy or transferred from sample to sample during RNA extractions can generate false-positives during the 100,000 or more public health rabies examinations conducted annually in laboratories in the United States. Furthermore, primer selection and the identification of truly universal primer sets for rabies and rabies-related viruses may still be a barrier to withholding rabies treatment based solely on negative PCR results.

DIAGNOSIS OF RABIES IN HUMANS

Because of the efficacy of modern cell culture vaccines and high-potency, purified human rabies immune globulin (HRIG), human rabies cases in the United States and other developed nations are no longer commonly associated with vaccine failure. Also, in these regions, rabies prophylaxis is provided in all cases of known, and even in most cases of suspected, exposure to rabies. Therefore, human cases are most often identified in the absence of a clear history of suspicious animal bite or other exposure. In numerous recent human rabies cases in the

United States, the disease was not suspected or diagnosed during the clinical illness and was recognized only postmortem, sometimes after a lengthy delay.[21]

There is great value in early recognition of human rabies infection to aid in patient management and initiation of postexposure treatment for potentially exposed family and caregivers and to prevent further avoidable exposures. Also, the recognition of all human rabies cases is very important in identification of highest risk exposure routes, vectors, and rabies virus variants. This information is essential to the development of effective rabies control and exposure management protocols. Therefore, antemortem rabies diagnosis should be attempted in all cases of acute, progressive human encephalitis of unknown etiology, even in the absence of a history of suspicious exposure.

Of course, brain biopsy would be the most sensitive antemortem diagnostic method, but because of the great risk of the procedure, it is not commonly used. Numerous less invasive intravitam tests can confirm rabies infection. However, rabies virus, its antigens, and rabies RNA do not move centrifugally away from the CNS during the incubation period and only slowly during the clinical period.[4] Humoral antibody responses similarly do not occur during the incubation period and are generally not demonstrable until the 2nd week of illness. Therefore, the sensitivity of antemortem diagnosis efforts is served by the analysis of numerous tissues by several methods, searching for viral antigen, rabies-specific antibody, live virus, and viral RNA.

Antigen detection can best be accomplished by FAT performed on a full thickness skin biopsy taken from the nape of the neck and including several hair follicles (Figure 4). FAT can also be used to demonstrate rabies antigen in corneal impression slides (Figure 5). Because of the risk of corneal abrasions, it is recommended that these samples be taken by an ophthalmologist.[24] Virus isolation by MIT or cell culture inoculation can be applied to saliva and cerebrospinal fluid (CSF). Antibody assay can be performed by neutralization test or indirect FAT on serum and CSF. Nested RT-PCR is applied to saliva. Demonstration of rabies antigen by FAT in any tissue, rabies RNA in saliva, rabies antibody in CSF, or isolation of rabies virus from any tissue is confirmatory of rabies infection. Antibody in serum alone may not be indicative of clinical rabies in a patient with known or unclear history of rabies vaccination or treatment with HRIG.

A review of 32 human rabies deaths in the United States from 1980 to 1996 disclosed that in 12 of the cases rabies was not suspected until after death. Of the remaining 20 cases, antemortem evidence of rabies was found by one or more tests in 18 cases. Antibody to rabies was detected in 10 of 18 tested, virus was isolated from saliva in 9 of 15 cases, and RNA was detected by PCR in each of the 10 tested by this means. Antigen was demonstrated by FAT in the skin in 10 of 15 tested, antigen in corneal impressions was present in 2 of 7 tested, and antigen was present in brain biopsy in all 3 examined in that manner.[21]

When human rabies is suspected, the laboratory should be contacted immediately. Samples should be collected for all currently used diagnostic procedures, and it must be remembered that repeat samples may be necessary because antemortem tests may remain negative well into the clinical period. The samples for antibody assay are 1 ml or more of CSF and serum. The skin biopsy can be submitted on a gauze sponge moistened with sterile physiologic saline and sealed in a small plastic container. Corneal impression slides should be submitted in a plastic slide container with the surface of the slide containing the impression clearly marked. A 1-ml sample of frank saliva should be collected into a plastic sputum jar. Alternatively, a buccal swab can be taken and submitted immersed in a tube

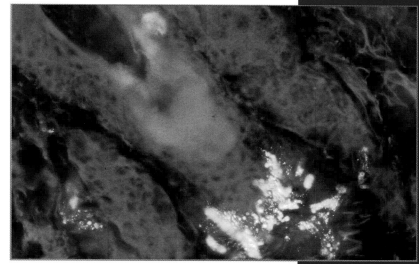

Figure 4—Rabies virus antigen in nerve cells at base of hair follicle in frozen section of skin. (Direct immunofluorescent staining with Evans blue counterstain, ×160.)

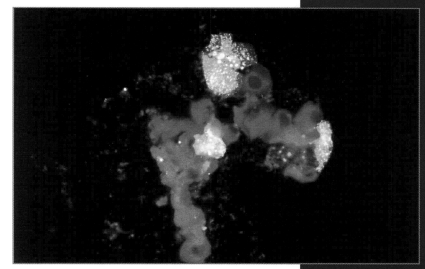

Figure 5—Rabies virus antigen in corneal impression. (Direct immunofluorescent staining with Evans blue counterstain, ×360.)

containing 1 ml of sterile saline. All of these samples can be stored at −70°C and shipped on dry ice. Postmortem testing methods for human rabies are similar to those described for animals. If the patient dies and an autopsy is performed, the ideal sample for

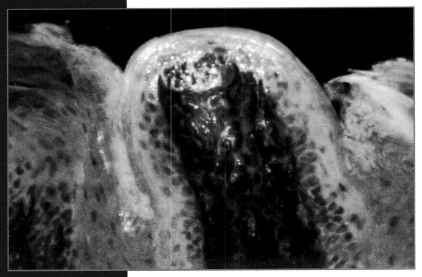

Figure 6—Direct immunofluorescent staining of rabies virus antigen in nerve cells in sensory papillae of tongue of silver-haired bat (Lasionycteris noctivagans) infected with the silver-haired/pipistrelle variant (×160).

postmortem diagnosis is 1-cm³ samples of unfixed cerebellum, brain stem, and hippocampus, preserved by refrigeration.

ANTEMORTEM DIAGNOSIS OF ANIMAL RABIES

The methods described for antemortem diagnosis of human rabies can be applied to suspect animals as well. Skin biopsy has been demonstrated to be particularly sensitive when applied to biopsies taken from the snout of terrestrial carnivores that permit examination of the innervation of the tactile hairs.[25] However, the same limitations apply to antemortem diagnosis in animals: Because all tests can remain negative well into or throughout the clinical period, negative results do not rule out rabies. Therefore, these tests are of little value for public health decisions and should never be a substitute when circumstances require 10-day observation or euthanasia and examination of brain tissue.

RABIES VIRUS VARIANT TYPING

The rabies virus variants responsible for the major terrestrial outbreaks worldwide, the numerous bat rabies variants, the laboratory strains of rabies virus, and the rabies-related strains of *Lyssavirus* are distinguished in the laboratory by their antigenic or genetic characteristics.

Reaction patterns in indirect FATs employing panels of monoclonal antibodies specific for unique viral nucleocapsid epitopes permit such discrimination.[26] The immunofluorescence assays can be performed on original case tissue or on mouse- or cell-culture-passaged virus. The identification of distinctive antigenic differences in this manner serves as an epidemiologic marker system for the study of variant prevalence and distribution and for the recognition of source of infection in individual cases (Fig. 6).

Genetic analysis permits more precise detail of the evolutionary relatedness of isolates, investigation of the spatial and temporal changes that may occur, and particularly the measure of similarity among virus isolates. This is accomplished by the extraction, transcription, and amplification of the RNA of an isolate by RT-PCR and the subsequent sequence analysis of the cDNA nucleotide or amino acid sequence for the entire or partial nucleocapsid or glycoprotein genes. Computer algorithms are used to perform pair-wise comparisons, calculating estimates of genetic identity expressed as percent homology among isolates.[27]

SUMMARY

Limitations of rabies diagnostic methods are determined by the unique pathogenesis of rabies infection and must be understood by clinicians. Rabies cannot be reliably diagnosed by current methods during most of the incubation period—claims that molecular testing of saliva of a biting animal can be used for decisions of bite management are false, as rabies virus may be shed in saliva sporadically prior to and during the clinical period.[4] Antemortem testing in animals and humans as described can reliably confirm rabies infection but cannot conclusively rule it out. However, the modern rabies laboratory can be a powerful tool to public health professionals in their rabies-control activities. Rabies infection in an animal can be confirmed or excluded with virtual 100% certainty by postmortem examination within hours of receipt of the specimen. Backup testing can be performed in vitro, providing timely confirmation of microscopic examination results and eliminating use of thousands of laboratory mice annually. Diagnostic reagents have been improved with the application of monoclonal antibody technology to FAT conjugates. Antemortem human rabies diagnosis has grown more sensitive with the addition of molecular methods to the existing battery of tests. Immunohistochemical analysis has been improved by tissue digestion and monoclonal antibodies, and along with molecular analysis, promises more sensitive analysis on formalin-fixed samples. Rabies virus variants can be identified simply for general epidemiologic analysis by panels of monoclonal antibodies and more precisely for evolutionary relationships by nucleotide sequence analysis. Clinicians should avail themselves of every benefit of collaboration with the laboratory by initiating contact with the local and central reference laboratories servicing their area to gain familiarity with laboratory policies, practices, and capabilities.

ACKNOWLEDGMENTS

The authors wish to thank Ms. Jean Smith and Dr. Charles Rupprecht of the Centers for Disease Control and Prevention and Mr. James Powell of the Wisconsin State Laboratory of Hygiene for their review and valuable comments to this chapter. We thank Dr. Alex Wandeler of the Canadian Food Inspection Agency for generously providing monoclonal antibody 5DF12, which was used as the first antibody for the immunohistochemical preparation for Figure 5.

REFERENCES

1. Centers for Disease Control and Prevention: Recommendations of the Advisory Committee on Immunization Practices (ACIP): Human rabies prevention—United States, 1999. *MMWR Morbid Mortal Wkly Rep* 48(RR-1):1–21, 1999.
2. Childs JE, Colby L, Krebs JW, et al: Surveillance and spatiotemporal associations of rabies in rodents and lagomorphs in the United States. *J Wildl Dis* 33(1):20–27, 1997.
3. Centers for Disease Control and Prevention: Human rabies—Montana and Washington, 1997. *MMWR Morbid Mortal Wkly Rep* 46(33):770–774, August 22, 1997.
4. Charlton KM: The pathogenesis of rabies, in Campbell JB, Charlton KM (eds): *Rabies.* Norwell, MA, Academic Press, 1988, pp 101–150.
5. Schleifstein J, Tompkins V: Rabies in cattle—A laboratory technique for removal of the cerebellum for laboratory examination. *JAVMA* 119(893): 130–132, 1951.
6. Barrat J: Simple technique for the collection and shipment of brain specimens for rabies diagnosis, in Meslin F-X, Kaplan MM, Koprowski H (eds): *Laboratory Techniques in Rabies,* ed 4. Geneva, World Health Organization, 1996, pp 425–432.
7. Perl DP, Good PF: The pathology of rabies in the central nervous system, in Baer GM (ed): *The Natural History of Rabies,* ed 2. Boca Raton, CRC Press, 1991, pp 163–190.
8. Tierkel ES, Atanasiu P: Rapid microscopic examination for Negri bodies and preparation of specimens for biological tests, in Meslin F-X, Kaplan MM, Koprowski H (eds): *Laboratory Techniques in Rabies,* ed 4. Geneva, World Health Organization, 1996, pp 55–65.
9. Lepine P, Atanasiu P: Histopathological diagnosis, in Meslin F-X, Kaplan MM, Koprowski H (eds): *Laboratory Techniques in Rabies,* ed 4. Geneva, World Health Organization, 1996, pp 66–79.
10. Trimarchi CV, Debbie JG: The fluorescent antibody in rabies, in Baer GM (ed): *The Natural History of Rabies,* ed 2. Boca Raton, CRC Press, 1991, pp 220–233.
11. Powell J: Proficiency testing in the rabies diagnostic laboratory. Abstracts of The Eighth Annual Rabies in the Americas Conference, Kingston, Ontario, November 2–6, 1997.
12. Report of the rabies diagnosis subcommittee of the Committee to Develop a Strategy to Control Rabies in the United States. CDC, October, 1994. In Press.
13. Rudd RJ, Trimarchi CV: The development and evaluation of an in vitro virus isolation procedure as a replacement for the mouse inoculation test in rabies diagnosis. *J Clin Microbiol* 27(11): 2522–2528, 1989.
14. Rudd RJ, Trimarchi CV: Tissue culture technique for routine isolation of street strain rabies virus. *J Clin Microbiol* 12(4):590–593, 1980.
15. Webster WA, Casey GA: Virus isolation in neuroblastoma cell culture, in Meslin F-X, Kaplan MM, Koprowski H (eds): *Laboratory Techniques in Rabies,* ed 4. Geneva, World Health Organization, 1996, pp 96–104.
16. Warner CK, Whitfield SG, Fekadu M, Ho H: Procedures for reproducible detection of rabies virus antigen, mRNA and genome in situ in formalin fixed tissues. *J Virol Methods* 67(1):5–12,1997.
17. Hamir AN, Moser ZF, Fu F, et al: Immunohistochemical test for rabies: Identification of a diagnostically superior monoclonal antibody. *Vet Rec* 136:295–296, 1995.

Rabies cannot be reliably diagnosed by current methods during most of the incubation period.

18. Bourhy H, Perrin P: Rapid rabies enzyme immunodiagnosis (RREID) for rabies antigen detection, in Meslin F-X, Kaplan MM, Koprowski H (eds): *Laboratory Techniques in Rabies*, ed 4. Geneva, World Health Organization, 1996, pp 105–113.

19. Tordo N, Bourhy H, Sacromento D: PCR technology for *Lyssavirus* diagnosis, in Clewly J (ed): *The Polymerase Chain Reaction (PCR) for Human Viral Diagnosis.* London, CRC Press, 1995, pp 125–145.

20. Kamolvarin N, Tirawatnpong T, Rattanasiwamoke R, et al: Diagnosis of rabies by polymerase chain reaction with nested primers. *J Infect Dis* 167:207–210, 1993.

21. Noah DL, Drenzek CL, Smith JS, et al: The epidemiology of human rabies in the United States, 1980–1996. *Ann Intern Med* 128:922–930, 1998.

22. Nadin-Davis SA, Huang W, Wandeler AI: The design of strain-specific polymerase chain reactions for discrimination of the raccoon rabies virus strain from indigenous rabies viruses of Ontario. *J Virol Meth* 57:141–156, 1996.

23. Smith JS: Rabies virus, in Murray PR, Baron EJ, Pfaller MA, et al (eds): *Manual of Clinical Microbiology,* ed 7. Washington, DC, ASM Press, 1999, pp 1099–1106.

24. Zaidman GW, Billingsly A: Corneal impression test for the diagnosis of acute rabies encephalitis. *Ophthalmology* 105:249–251, 1998.

25. Blenden DC, Bell JF, Tsao AT, Umoh JV: Immunofluorescent examination of the skin of rabies infected animals as a means of early detection of rabies virus antigen. *J Clin Microbiol* 18:631–636, 1983.

26. Smith JS, Reid-Sanden FL, Roumillat LF, et al: Demonstration of antigen variation among rabies virus isolates by using monoclonal antibodies to nucleocapsid proteins. *J Clin Microbiol* 24(4):573–580, 1986.

27. Smith JS, Orciari LA, Yager PA, et al: Epidemiologic and historical relationships among 87 rabies virus isolates as determined by limited sequence analysis. *J Infect Dis* 166:296–307, 1992.

Rabies Vaccines

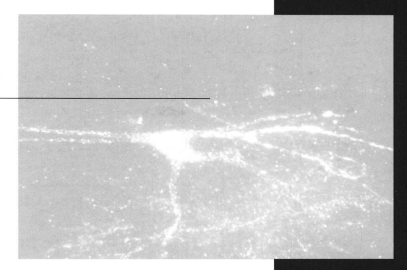

Kent R. Van Kampen, DVM, PhD
Diplomate ACVP
CEO, The Van Kampen Group, Inc.
Ogden, Utah

HISTORICAL ASPECTS

Vaccination has been the major means of controlling rabies since 1881 when Galtier[1] at the veterinary school in Lyon, France, first initiated the protection of sheep and goats against rabies by inoculating them with the saliva taken from a rabid animal. In 1884, following the lead of Galtier, Louis Pasteur and colleagues[2] made preparations of the spinal cords of rabbits that had died of rabies and injected this material into a series of dogs. Upon subsequent challenge with virulent rabies virus, the dogs were protected against rabies. Later, Pasteur attempted to save the life of a 9-year-old boy, Joseph Meister, who had been severely bitten by a rabid dog several days earlier. The young boy was injected daily for 11 days with a series of Pasteur's spinal cord preparation from rabbits. Miraculously, the young boy survived.

VACCINATION AND VACCINES

Even with the scientific knowledge to combat rabies, vaccination did not become well established until early in the 20th century. Reservoirs[3] for this deadly disease have existed worldwide in various wildlife populations including wolves, coyotes, foxes, raccoons, skunks, bats, mongooses, jackals, raccoon dogs, and feral populations of dogs and cats. Exposure of humans to rabies was usually due to a bite by one of these rabid wild animals or by a domestic animal that had become infected by a bite from a wild animal. Japanese veterinarians[4] first attempted to bring the disease under control by vaccinating dogs in a countrywide program. Their pioneering program was interrupted by World War II, but it was reinitiated thereafter and continued to be very successful.[5] It was not until 1946 that veterinarians in North America[6] and in Europe began to actively recommend that dogs be vaccinated against rabies. Since that time, the number of cases of rabies in dogs, and subsequently in people, has dramatically decreased. A protective barrier against rabies has been created by the widespread immunization of companion animals, primarily dogs and cats.

Vaccines of various types have been used for the immunization of humans and domestic animals. The earlier vaccines were made from rabies-infected animals from which nervous tissue[7] was obtained and treated with formalin, ether, or other substances to kill the virus. Sheep, goats, rabbits, and mice served as the sources of the nervous tissue. Suckling mouse brain[8] continues to be used as a substrate for rabies vaccine in some countries. Duck and chicken embryos[9,10] were

A protective barrier against rabies has been created by the widespread immunization of companion animals, primarily dogs and cats.

The advent of

tissue culture

vaccines replicated

on specific cell

lines has led to

the widespread

use of rabies

vaccines

throughout the

world.

used to grow rabies virus for vaccine use, but the unpurified antigen caused significant allergic reactions. Modified live rabies vaccines have been used in some countries to vaccinate pets, but the possibility of reversion to virulence remains an issue with these vaccines. The advent of tissue culture vaccines replicated on specific cell lines has led to the widespread use of rabies vaccines throughout the world, in both humans and animals. These vaccines have been demonstrated to be highly antigenic, safe, and economical for use in animals worldwide. One of these, Imrab® (Merial), has been licensed in the United States for the vaccination of six different animal species including dogs, cats, cattle, horses, sheep, and ferrets. Duration of immunity ranges from 1 to 3 years, depending on the species in which the vaccine is used. Because of the protective barrier provided by vaccination against rabies of companion and domestic animals, human exposure to rabies today is significantly less than earlier in the 20th century.

COMPENDIUM OF ANIMAL RABIES CONTROL[11]

Immunization procedures for animals to be vaccinated against rabies in the United States are updated annually in a document titled *Compendium of Animal Rabies Control,* (year of issue [i.e., *1999*]), found on page 79 of this book. These recommendations are provided to ensure that veterinarians are informed about the current requirements, regulations, and products that govern or provide for immunization of domestic and wild animals. The document is divided into three main sections: Part I: Recommendations for Parenteral Immunization Procedures; Part II: Rabies Vaccines Licensed in the USA and NASPHV (National Association of State Public Health Veterinarians), recommendations for that particular year; and Part III: Rabies Control.

Part I includes sections on vaccine administration, vaccine selection, route of inoculation, vaccination of wildlife and hybrids, accidental human exposures to the vaccines, and identification of animals known to carry rabies. The *Compendium* designates the adoption of a standard tagging system for animals vaccinated against rabies that includes a color and shape coding corresponding to the particular year that the animal was immunized. It also recommends that a certificate of rabies vaccination be issued to the animal's owner at the time of immunization.

Part II lists all of the rabies vaccines currently licensed in the United States and gives the product name, the manufacturer, the marketer, the species for which the vaccine is licensed, the dosage, the age requirement for primary immunization, recommendations for boosters, and the route of inoculation. Most rabies vaccines for dogs and cats are administered at 3 months of age, boosted at 1 year of age, and thereafter given triennially via either the intramuscular or the subcutaneous route of administration. Depending on the vaccine, rabies vaccines for livestock may be administered annually or triennially following primary inoculation.

Part III deals with the principles of rabies control, control methods in domestic and confined animals as well as other animals, including preexposure vaccination, quarantine procedures, licensure, postexposure management, and control methods in wildlife.

RECOMBINANT VACCINES

With the advent of genetic engineering and the understanding of the genetic code, many microorganisms, both pathogenic and nonpathogenic, have been studied to the point that many of their genetic secrets have been unmasked. Genes associated with virulence, pathogenicity, host range, structural proteins, and antigens that invoke protective immunity have been isolated and sequenced. The glycoprotein from the outer surface of the rabies virus has been demonstrated to provoke a protective antibody response against all known variants of the rabies virus. With the isolation of the gene encoding the rabies glycoprotein by the Wistar Institute, the potential of creating a recombinant vaccine has become possible.

In 1978, Dr. Enzo Paoletti and his associates (internal documents) at the New York State Health Department's Wadsworth Laboratories developed a technology using the smallpox vaccine, vaccinia, as a vector to introduce extraneous genetic material to the immune system. This was accomplished by eliminating some of the genes from the vaccinia virus and inserting foreign DNA (taken from another organism) into the vaccinia virus by recombination. Using this technology, Jean Pierre Lecocq[12] and his team at Transgene in France interrupted the thymidine kinase gene by removing DNA from the vaccinia virus and at that site inserted the gene taken from the rabies virus, which encoded the glycoprotein. When this recombinant virus was tested in mice by injection, it was found to invoke a protective antibody response against a lethal challenge of rabies virus. Subsequent tests demonstrated that a similar protective response could be obtained in animals if the virus was injected subcutaneously, intramuscularly, or intradermally. What surprised the researchers was that when the recombinant vaccine was administered orally, a similar protection against a rabies challenge was noted.[13] Based on earlier experience of scientists using a modified live viral vaccine,[14] Swiss and Canadian officials placed the modified live rabies vaccine strains SAD or ERA into chicken heads or into tallow baits, which were then used to protect foxes against rabies. This experience led to the conclusion that this recombinant vaccine should be tested as a wildlife vaccine.

Today, this recombinant viral vaccine has been used successfully and safely[15,16] to orally vaccinate a variety of wild animal species against rabies. Early studies in France and Belgium demonstrated that the vaccine could be placed in baits that would be eaten by red foxes. A fishmeal polymer bait was developed that was rectangular in shape with a hollow chamber to receive the vaccine container. The vaccine was placed in plastic sachets, inserted into the hollow chamber of the bait, and secured by wax. Because the vaccinia virus was stable at a wide range of ambient temperatures,[17] the vaccine remained viable for up to 30 days after the baits were placed in the habitat of the foxes.

Beginning in 1989, the recombinant vaccine-bait combination was released by aerial distribution into the enzootic rabies habitat of the red fox along the Franco-Belgian border. Over a 5-year period, with a spring and autumn distribution of baits containing vaccine, rabies as a disease was virtually eliminated from that area.[18] Testing of the vaccine in the United States proceeded with programs to immunize raccoons, coyotes, and gray foxes. Research efforts[19–21] demonstrated that the vaccine could be used (1) to create a geographical barrier wherein the immunization of raccoons prevented an epizootic of rabies from progressing into a rabies-free area, (2) to reduce rabies infection in a wildlife population experiencing an epizootic of rabies, and (3) to control the spread of rabies within an area with enzootic rabies infection in the wildlife population. Oral Rabies Vaccination Programs (ORVPs) in Texas have been highly effective in controlling rabies in coyotes and gray foxes.[22] In 1997, the United States Department of Agriculture licensed the oral recombinant Raboral V-RG (Merial) for use in control of rabies in raccoons.

Dr. Paoletti's group has created three viral vectors from the poxviruses for commercial use in vaccine[23]:

■ TROVAC® (Virogenetics) is a fowlpox vector used for recombinant poultry vaccines such as avian influenza and Newcastle disease.
■ NYVAC® (Virogenetics) is a multiple gene–deleted vaccinia used experimentally for a number of vaccines for domestic animals.

With the isolation of the gene encoding the rabies glycoprotein, the potential of creating a recombinant vaccine has become possible.

■ ALVAC® (Virogenetics) is a gene-deleted, host-restricted canarypox vector used for vaccines in companion animals. The canarypox vector is unable to replicate when exposed to mammalian cells and is therefore an ideal vector because it will not be transmitted from animal to animal or shed into the environment.

New recombinant canarypox-vectored canine distemper and rabies vaccines[24] have been licensed and introduced for use in companion animals. These nonadjuvanted vaccines have been demonstrated to be very safe and convey a solid protective immunity.

Influence of Maternal Antibodies

While experimenting with the vaccinia recombinant used for vaccinating wildlife, researchers injected this vaccine into 2-week-old puppies born to bitches previously vaccinated against rabies. Some littermates were not vaccinated. At 419 days after vaccination, these dogs were challenged with rabies virus.[24] The nonvaccinates succumbed to rabies, while those vaccinated at 2 weeks of age were solidly protected. It has always been accepted that immunity against rabies could not be achieved while puppies had circulating levels of passive or maternally transferred rabies antibodies.

Subsequent to this experiment, a study designed to follow the maternal antibody level in puppies born to bitches hyperimmunized against rabies with either a canarypox recombinant rabies vaccine or a conventional tissue culture rabies vaccine (Imrab) demonstrated that passive antibody remained high until the sixth week, at which time it began to decline, so that by 12 weeks of age none of the puppies had circulating maternal antibody against rabies.

In a similar study, groups of puppies born to bitches hyperimmunized against rabies with the canarypox recombinant or the conventional Imrab were divided into three groups. One group was immunized with a single injection of Imrab at 6 weeks of age, one group was immunized with a single injection of canarypox rabies recombinant at 6 weeks of age, and one group was unimmunized. Additionally, puppies born to non–rabies-vaccinated bitches were divided into three groups. One group was immunized with a single injection of Imrab at 6 weeks of age, one group was immunized with a single injection of canarypox rabies recombinant at 6 weeks of age, and one group was not immunized. At 4 months of age, all of the puppies were challenged with virulent rabies virus. All of the puppies that had been immunized with either the Imrab or the canarypox rabies recombinant survived the challenge, while the nonvaccinated puppies succumbed to the challenge.[24] None of the puppies injected with either vaccine at 6 weeks of age demonstrated a significant rise in antibody titer until after the challenge. Yet all were solidly protected, primarily because sufficient memory cells had been created by the immune system to create an immunity upon challenge. This means that puppies can be immunized against rabies at a much earlier age than previously had been thought. This may lead to new recommendations for vaccination of puppies prior to 12 weeks of age.

Experimental Approaches

Other vectors have been used experimentally to create rabies vaccines. Extensive work has taken place using adenoviruses[25] as a recombinant vector. Although this vector can effectively deliver the rabies glycoprotein gene, it is often shed or transmitted from the vaccinate into the environment or to other animals. Plasmid DNA preparations[26] have been used in mice to convey genes from the rabies virus. Mice vaccinated in this manner have been protected against rabies.[27] In a limited study at the Public Health Laboratory in Hamilton, Montana, monkeys were also protected using this approach. Work has also taken place to transfer the rabies glycoprotein gene into plants.[28] Consumption of these plants results in a low-level protection. Purification of the glycoprotein from the plant and subsequent injection into mice will protect the mice against rabies.

SUMMARY

Vaccination is a cost-effective means of protecting companion animals and livestock against rabies. Safe and efficacious vaccines exist to vaccinate animals and humans by provoking an immunologic response that is strongly protective. New recombinant vaccines have been developed using poxvirus vectors that are now licensed for use in companion animals. The vaccinia rabies recombinant Raboral V-RG has been used to orally vaccinate wildlife by combining the vaccine with an edible bait that can be distributed into the habitat of the target animal species. New studies indicate that maternal antibody against rabies may interfere with antibody production upon vaccination of 6-week-old puppies, yet the puppies are solidly protected against an otherwise lethal challenge of rabies virus. Look for earlier immunization recommendations for puppies.

REFERENCES

1. Galtier V: Etudes sur la rage. *Ann Med Vet* 28: 627–639, 1879.
2. Pasteur L, Chamberland C, Roux E: Sur la rage. *Bull Acad Natl Med* 25:661–664, 1884.
3. Fu ZF: Rabies and rabies research: Past, present and future. *Vaccine* 15 (Suppl):S20–S24, 1997.
4. Umeno S, Soi YA: A Study on the anti-rabic inoculation of dogs and the results of its practical application. *Arch Exp Med (Kitisato)* 4:89–102, 1921.
5. Smidada K, in Nagano Y, Davenport FM (eds): *The Last Rabies Outbreak in Japan.* Baltimore, University Park Press, 1971.
6. Johnson HN: Experimental and Field Studies of Canine Rabies Vaccination. Baltimore, Proceedings of the 49th Annual Meeting of the US Livestock Sanitary Association, 1946.
7. Dreesen DW: A global review of rabies vaccines for human use. *Vaccine* 15 (Suppl):S2–S6, 1997.
8. Fuenzalida E, Palacio R: Rabies vaccine prepared from the brains of infected suckling mice. *Boletin del Instiututo Backeriologico de Chile* 8:3–10, 1955.
9. Peck FB, Powell HM, Culbertson CB: Duck embryo rabies vaccine. Study of fixed virus vaccine grown in embryonating duck eggs and killed with beta-propiolactone. *JAMA* 162:1373–1376, 1956.
10. Beveridge, Burnett FM: The cultivation of viruses and rickettsiae in the chick embryo. *MRC Special Report Series #256.* HMSO London, 1946.
11. *Compendium of Animal Rabies Control, 1998.* Copyright by the American Veterinary Medical Association, 1998.
12. Kieny MP, Lathe R, Drillien R, et al: Expression of rabies virus glycoprotein from a recombinant vaccinia virus. *Nature* 313:163–165, 1984.
13. Rupprecht CE, Wiktor TJ, Johnston D, et al: Oral immunization and protection of raccoons *(Procyon lotor)* with a vaccinia-rabies glycoprotein recombinant vaccinia virus vaccine. *Proc Natl Acad Sci U S A* 83:7947, 1986.
14. Baer GM, Abelseth MK, Debbie JG: Oral vaccination of foxes against rabies. *Am J Epidemiol* 93:487–489, 1971.
15. Pastoret PP, Brochier B: The development and use of a vaccinia-rabies recombinant oral vaccine for the control of wildlife rabies; a link between Jenner and Pasteur. *Epidemiol Infect* 116(3):235–240, 1996.
16. Hanlon CA, Niezgoda M, Hamir AN, et al: First North American field release of a vaccinia-rabies glycoprotein recombinant virus. *J Wildl Dis* 34(2):228–239, 1998.
17. Pastoret PP, Brochier B, Languet B, et al: Stability of recombinant vaccinia-rabies vaccine in veterinary use. *Dev Biol Stand* 87:245–249, 1996.
18. Brochier B, Costy F, Pastoret PP: Elimination of fox rabies from Belgium using a recombinant vaccinia-rabies vaccine: An update. *Vet Microbiol* 46(1–3):269–279, 1995.
19. Hable CP, Hamir AN, Snyder DE, et al: Prerequisites for oral immunization of free-ranging raccoons *(Procyon lotor)* with a recombinant rabies virus vaccine: Study site ecology and bait system development. *J Wildl Dis* 28:64–79, 1992.
20. Robbins A, Rowell S, Bordon M, et al: Update on the Prevention of Rabies Spread by Oral Vaccination of Raccoons on Cape Cod, Massachusetts. Kingston, Ontario, Canada, Eighth Annual Rabies in the Americas Conference, November 2–6, 1997.
21. Willsey A: The New York State Department of Health Oral Wildlife Rabies Vaccination Studies. Kingston, Ontario, Canada, Eighth Annual Rabies in the Americas Conference, November 2–6, 1997.
22. Fearneyhough MG: Summary of the Texas Oral Rabies Vaccination Program. Kingston, Ontario, Canada, Eighth Annual Rabies in the Americas Conference, November 2–6, 1997.
23. Paoletti E: Applications of pox virus vectors to vaccination: An update. *Proc Natl Acad Sci U S A* 93(21):11349–11353, 1996.
24. Merial: Data on file.
25. Yarosh OK, Wandler AI, Graham FL, et al: Human adenovirus type 5 vectors expressing rabies glycoprotein. *Vaccine* 14(13):1257–1264, 1996.
26. Wang Y, Ziang Z, Pasquinit S, Ertl HC: Immune responses to neonatal genetic immunization. *Virology* 228(2):278–284, 1997.
27. Ray NB, Ewalt LC, Lodmell DL: Nanogram quantities of plasmid DNA encoding the rabies virus glycoprotein protected mice against lethal rabies virus infection. *Vaccine* 15(8):892–895, 1997.
28. McGarvey PB, Hammond J, Dienelt MM, et al: Expression of the rabies virus glycoprotein in transgenic tomatoes. *Biotechnology* 13:1484–1487, 1995.

The vaccinia rabies recombinant Raboral V-RG has been used to orally vaccinate wildlife by combining the vaccine with an edible bait that can be distributed into the habitat of the target animal species.

Importation of Dogs and Cats to Rabies-Free Areas of the World

Deborah J. Briggs, PhD
Professor/Director, Rabies Laboratory
Kansas State University College of Veterinary Medicine
Manhattan, Kansas

Public pressure from a very mobile society has caused the governments of many rabies-free areas to reevaluate their quarantine system.

THE WORLD HEALTH ORGANIZATION (WHO) DEFINES A RABIES-FREE AREA AS "ONE IN WHICH AN EFFECTIVE IMPORT POLICY IS IMPLEMENTED AND, IN THE PRESENCE OF ADEQUATE DISEASE SURVEILLANCE, NO CASE OF INDIGENOUSLY ACQUIRED RABIES INFECTION HAS BEEN CONFIRMED IN HUMANS OR ANY ANIMAL SPECIES AT ANY TIME DURING THE PREVIOUS TWO YEARS."[1] THE PRESENCE OR ABSENCE OF RABIES VIRUS IN THE INDIGENOUS BAT POPULATION IS NOT INCLUDED IN THE WHO DEFINITION. COUNTRIES AND AREAS WHERE NO RABIES WAS REPORTED IN 1996 ARE PUBLISHED AT THE WHO WORLD WIDE WEB SITE (WWW.WHO.INT/EMC/DISEASES/ZOO/RABNET.HTML) AND INCLUDE BUT ARE NOT LIMITED TO AUSTRALIA, BAHAMAS, FIJI, FINLAND, GREECE, HAWAII, HONG KONG, ICELAND, JAPAN, NEW ZEALAND, PAPUA NEW GUINEA, PORTUGAL, ST. KITTS-NEVIS, SINGAPORE, SWEDEN, AND THE UNITED KINGDOM.

Prior to the advent of highly efficacious killed rabies vaccines, lengthy quarantine laws for dogs and cats entering rabies-free areas were used as a means of preventing the introduction or reintroduction of rabies. However, quarantine periods of 4 to 6 months have become increasingly unacceptable to many people relocating to rabies-free areas who wish to take their family pets with them. Resultant public pressure from a very mobile society has caused the governments of many rabies-free areas to reevaluate their quarantine system. In the Eighth Report of the WHO Expert Committee on Rabies, alternate recommendations to lengthy quarantine requirements were made that would continue to ensure the protection of rabies-free areas while simultaneously reducing the length of time required for a dog or cat to be held in a quarantine facility.[1] Several rabies-free areas have embraced all or part of the WHO recommendations, while others are in the process of reviewing or updating their import requirements for dogs and cats from countries in which rabies is present but well controlled. Rabies-free areas that have replaced their lengthy quarantine periods for dogs and cats being imported from the United States with alternate measures include Australia, New Zealand, St. Kitts-Nevis, and Hawaii. Between 1995 and 1998, more than 15,000 dogs and cats have been imported into these areas with no reports of rabies being introduced or re-introduced.

When preparing to move to a rabies-free area that has strict importation regulations regarding dogs and cats, meeting the criteria to qualify for a reduced quarantine program requires time, patience, and advanced preparation. Several commercial companies specialize in pet moving services, relieving the owner of the tedious and often complicated preparation that is necessary to fulfill governmental requirements. If a pet relocation specialist is chosen by the owner to help with the move, the specialist should be reputable and should preferably belong to the Independent Pet and Animal Transport Association International, Inc. (IPATA). Members of the IPATA are registered or licensed by the United States Department of Agriculture (USDA) (in the United States) and form a network of pet shippers throughout the world. If pet owners decide to forgo the services of a pet relocation service, they should contact the consulate of the destination country well in advance of anticipated departure to determine the regulations required for importing their animal. In addition, they should work with their veterinarian to assist with the preparations for moving their pet. It is critical to review and understand the importation regulations that the rabies-free areas have in place. For example, some rabies-free countries prohibit the importation of certain breeds of dogs and cats and, even if all other requirements have been fulfilled and the animal arrives in the destination country, entry will be denied. The owner will be responsible for removing the animal from the country or, in a worst-case scenario, the animal will be destroyed.

REQUIREMENTS

The requirements for dogs and cats entering rabies-free areas can generally be obtained through the department of agriculture in the country in question or through its governmental consulate in Washington,

DC. Most countries require an import permit at some point in the importation process. Other requirements differ according to the country's specific laws, put in place to prevent the introduction or reintroduction of rabies (Table 1). Once the date of departure is determined by the owner, a calendar of tasks and required completion dates should be devised. The schedule for specific laboratory tests, examinations, and other treatments differs for each country, and inadvertently missing one of the target dates can delay an animal from being allowed entry into the destination country.

In general, most rabies-free areas require more blood tests to be conducted on dogs (i.e., *Brucella canis, Ehrlichia canis, Leptospira canicola,* microfilariae, and others) than on cats. In addition, at least four rabies-free areas require one or more rabies virus neutralization tests for both dogs and cats. All blood samples must be sent to a reference laboratory approved by the government of the destination area. If the animal is required to have an identifying microchip or tattoo in place, this must be accomplished prior to having the blood withdrawn. In addition, the date that the blood sample was drawn and the identifying microchip or tattoo number must be on the blood sample and the accompanying paperwork. Currently, Hawaii accepts only the AVID® (American Veterinary Identification Devices) microchips issued by the Hawaiian state governmental authorities. Australia and New Zealand require an official USDA veterinarian to sign all paperwork prior to the animal's leaving the country. Hawaii and St. Kitts-Nevis require the official laboratory to send the results directly to the governmental office in their state or country.

Rabies virus neutralization assays measure the animal's humoral immune response after vaccination. When the test is required, it is necessary to have a response of at least 0.5 IU/ml of rabies neutralizing antibody. The level of 0.5 IU/ml was originally select-

Most rabies-free areas require more blood tests to be conducted on dogs than on cats.

TABLE 1

Major Requirements for Dogs and Cats Entering Rabies-Free Zones from the United States[a]

Destination	Import Permit	Identification	Age Restriction	Rabies Vaccination	VNA[b] Test	Other Requirements
Australia	Yes	Microchip, health certificate	6 months or older	Yes	Yes	Some canine breeds not allowed entry. Additional tests and treatment required for dogs and cats to qualify for 30-day quarantine.
Bahamas	Yes	Health certificate	No	Yes	No	No quarantine.
Bermuda	Yes	Health certificate	No	Yes	No	Additional treatment required. No quarantine.
Finland	No	Health certificate	No	Yes	No	
Greece	No	Health certificate	No	Yes	No	No quarantine requirements.
Hawaii	No	Microchip, health certificate	Yes	Yes	Yes	Microchip must be issued by the state of Hawaii. Additional treatments and vaccinations required to qualify for 30-day quarantine.
Hong Kong	Yes	Health certificate	5 months or older	Yes	No	No quarantine for pets over 5 months of age. Must arrive as manifested air cargo.
Iceland	Yes	Health certificate	No	Yes	No	
Japan	No	Health certificate for dogs	No	Yes	No	Quarantine period for dogs is dependent upon rabies vaccination. No quarantine for cats.
New Zealand	Yes	Microchip or tattoo, health certificate	9 months or older	Yes	Yes	Some canine breeds not allowed entry. Additional tests and treatment required for dogs and cats to qualify for 30-day quarantine.
St. Kitts-Nevis	Yes	Microchip, health certificate	Yes	Yes	Yes	Must have had two rabies vaccinations at least 6 months apart. 30-day quarantine for dogs and cats that meet requirements.
Singapore	Yes	Health certificate	No	Yes	No	30-day quarantine in effect.
Sweden	Yes	Health certificate	No	Yes	No	4-month quarantine in effect.
United Kingdom	Yes	Health certificate	No	No	No	Current 6-month quarantine is under review.

[a]These requirements are subject to change; other requirements may apply.
[b]Virus neutralization antibody.

ed as the point at which nonspecific interference factors present in some serum samples no longer interfered with the neutralization of the rabies virus. In other words, when a rabies virus neutralizing antibody level of at least 0.5 IU/ml is present in the serum sample after vaccination, it is due to the fact that the animal has responded to the rabies antigen in the vaccine by producing neutralizing antibody, and it is not due to the presence of lipids or other serum factors that may neutralize the control rabies virus used in the assay. The question as to what level of rabies neutralizing antibody is required to protect a dog or cat has received much debate.[2,3] Study data indicate that some vaccinated animals with titers above 0.5 IU/ml may not survive a challenge with rabies virus, while some vaccinated animals with titers below 0.5 IU/ml may survive a similar challenge.[2] The reason that rabies neutralizing antibody titers should not be

TABLE 2
Information That Should Be Obtained from the Airline Carrier prior to Travel

- Airline carrier restrictions (container size, quantity of animals)
- Route of travel and whether the container will fit on all of the aircraft necessary for travel
- Time of arrival at the airport prior to departure
- Document requirements and other handling/shipping requirements with the airline (some carriers have restrictions for pug-nosed breeds of dogs and cats that are more stringent than USDA rules)
- Hours/days of customs and health facilities
- Location to drop off and pick up the animal
- Mode of transportation of the animal, that is, baggage or manifested freight
- Restrictions for unaccompanied pets (manifested freight)
- Restrictions on the size and number of animals allowed to travel in the cabin

correlated to protection against challenge is because rabies neutralization assays do not take into consideration the fact that cellular immunity is also involved in successfully surviving a challenge with rabies virus. Therefore, in the United States, there is no level of rabies neutralizing antibody that is considered "protective." However, rabies virus neutralization assays are a valuable tool in measuring whether an animal responded to a rabies vaccination and in some cases have identified animals that have an underlying immunosuppressive condition that prevents them from responding adequately to rabies vaccines.[4]

Two rabies virus neutralization assays are recognized by the Office des International Epizooties (OIE), the World Organization for Animal Health.[5] The rapid fluorescent focus inhibition test (RFFIT) and the fluorescent antibody virus neutralization (FAVN) test. Rabies-free areas, with the exception of the state of Hawaii, accept the results from either test. Hawaii will accept serologic results only from the FAVN test. Rabies-free areas may require more than one serologic test to be performed prior to entry and some require an additional test to be performed once the animal has landed in the rabies-free area. The consulate of the respective rabies-free area should be contacted for specific requirements. The RFFIT and the FAVN are based on the same principle and produce similar results on duplicate serum samples.[6]

SHIPPING REGULATIONS

When traveling from the mainland United States to a rabies-free area, it is necessary to make the journey in an airplane or an ocean-going vessel. The fastest and most humane method of transporting animals long distances is by air. However, not all airports in rabies-free areas have adequate facilities to accept animals. Therefore, it is necessary to contact the consulate of the destination country for airport customs information. To ensure that the animal arrives safely in the destination country, several factors (as outlined in Table 2) should be taken into consideration prior to booking the animal's flight.

The International Air Transport Association (IATA) Live Animals Regulations are recognized as the world standard for transporting animals by commercial airlines. However, some countries have more stringent standards than the IATA and should be contacted to clarify their requirements for shipping live animals. The IATA Live Animals Regulations include detailed information for choosing an appropriate shipping container and for safeguarding the welfare of the animals during the shipping process. The container requirements mandated by the IATA are based on the species and size of the animal(s). The size requirement for animal containers was carefully determined to prevent injury during travel while allowing the animal to travel in comfort. For short trips with small animals traveling in

In the United States, there is no level of rabies neutralizing antibody that is considered "protective."

75

the cabin with their owner, a soft carrying bag container is sufficient. For animals traveling in the hold, the container must be rigid and conform to the IATA Live Animals Regulations. It must be big enough for the animal to stand normally, turn around, and lie down. Air kennels must have the correct amount of ventilation openings for good air circulation during any flight. The airline should be contacted for assistance in determining the correct size. The container should be purchased ahead of time to allow the animal to become accustomed to it before travel. It is also advisable to feed the animal inside the container so that it takes "ownership" of the space.

As part of the initial preparations, the most appropriate route of travel needs to be selected. As mentioned previously, some airports do not have adequate facilities to handle the animal's needs. To coordinate days and times when the customs officers are on duty, it is important to consider the day of dispatch and the day of arrival. It is the responsibility of the shipper to make sure that all of the required documentation has been obtained and is securely attached to the airway bill. The shipper must provide the airline with two copies of the Shipper's Certification for Live Animals. The number and species of animals must also be stated on the airway bill. The airline that has been chosen to transport the pet should be contacted to determine whether they will accept the pet on the selected day and flight. The airline must be contacted a minimum of 48 hours in advance of departure to ensure that space is available for the animal. Small dogs and cats may or may not be allowed to travel in the cabin. If cabin travel is prohibited and the animal can travel as special cargo, it will be placed in a heated and ventilated hold.

Some airlines restrict the number of animals that they carry on any one flight, so advance reservations are strongly recommended. The length of check-in time required for the pet should be determined. If

the pet is traveling with the owner in the cabin and may become stressed in the airport crowds, such stress can be kept to a minimum by checking in as late as possible. If the animal will be traveling in the hold, the owner should check it in early so that it can go to the baggage area and relax in a quiet and dimly lit area. The food, *but not water*, intake should be reduced the day prior to travel. Dogs should be taken for a walk prior to setting out for the airport and if possible again before checking in. This will allow the animal to urinate and defecate prior to boarding. A light meal two hours prior to departure may help calm the animal, but it is unwise to feed it a heavy meal. If the animal is being shipped as air freight, the shipper should confirm that the air freight facility is open so that the animal may be claimed when it arrives. Weekdays are preferable to weekends for shipping because all staff are working and liaison is relatively easy along the route.

It is not advisable to ship animals (especially snub-nosed dogs) in the heat of the summer. The USDA requires that no more than two live puppies or kittens 8 weeks to 6 months of age, of comparable size, and weighing 20 lb or less be transported in the same primary enclosure. Even animals that share the same household may become stressed and aggressive toward each other when traveling by air. Food and water containers accessible from outside the container are required by the IATA. In addition, the airline carrier may require that supplemental food be provided in a pouch attached to the container with feeding instructions.

Some airlines will not accept animals handled by anyone other than a shipper, and therefore it may be necessary to hire an animal shipper who can make all of the necessary reservations and take full charge of the pet for the owner. If the animal is to be shipped as cargo, the owner should contact the airline for the time and date of the flight. The pet should be placed in the container and taken to the cargo department of the airline from 2 to 4 hours prior to departure. An airway bill must be filled out with the description of the animal and the total weight and dimensions of the container with the animal inside. The container must be correctly labeled with the standard IATA Live Animals Label and "This Way Up" labels on at least three sides of the container. The name and address of the owner, a 24-hour contact phone number, and the consignee's name and address must also be clearly fixed to the top of the container. Dried food must be supplied and written instructions for feeding and watering must be attached to the container in case there is a delay. In addition, any medication that has been or is being given must be recorded with the name of the drug and the route and time of administration.

Tranquilizers are not recommended for animals traveling via air. Drugs can have different reactions at pressures above 8,000 feet, and there is no way to determine how an animal will react. Finally, prior to shipment, reservations at quarantine facilities (if quarantine is required) should be made and the owner should have a clear understanding as to how and when the animal will be transported to these facilities.

FUTURE DIRECTIONS

A new era in rabies prevention was initiated in 1992 when the WHO Expert Committee on Rabies recommended alternate procedures to replace lengthy quarantine periods for dogs and cats entering rabies-free areas. Australia and New Zealand were the first countries to implement reduced quarantine procedures, followed a few years later by Hawaii and St. Kitts-Nevis. Although the reduced quarantine programs in these rabies-free areas are relatively new, they have received worldwide attention and to date have been very successful. The new quarantine programs depend upon positive identification through microchips or tattoos, documented rabies vaccinations, sero-

logic testing, and health certificates. If the programs instituted in these countries continue to be successful, and there is no reason to think that they will not be, increased pressure will be put on other rabies-free areas to follow their example.

In 1998 a panel of experts headed by Professor Ian Kennedy met in Great Britain to reevaluate rabies and the quarantine regulations that had been in place in that country for almost a century. The experts concluded that if dogs and cats were allowed to travel from Great Britain to the European Union (EU), to European Economic Area (EEA) member states, or to rabies-free islands and back again, there would be only a marginal increase in the already small risk of reintroducing rabies. In light of these findings, the committee recommended that certain dogs and cats that were residents of Great Britain be exempt from quarantine upon return from other EU, EEA, or rabies-free islands. In addition, the Kennedy committee recommended that further studies be conducted on the number of dogs and cats that would be imported from North America if the current quarantine system were not applied and also suggested that a risk assessment be conducted. If quarantine changes are implemented for North America, they will be the most radical and sweeping changes that have ever occurred in Great Britain's quarantine laws.

The forecast for the replacement of archaic quarantine systems is indeed bright. However, when rabies-free areas relax their rigorous quarantine laws, those laws must be replaced by vigilant importation requirements. Certified laboratories and federally licensed veterinarians need to work closely with the government officials of rabies-free areas to ensure that documentation is accurate and that potentially infected dogs and cats are identified and prevented from entering the country. Only under these circumstances will risk factors remain low and residents of rabies-free areas be assured that

When rabies-free areas relax their rigorous quarantine laws, those laws must be replaced by vigilant importation requirements.

rabies will not be reintroduced into their country.

REFERENCES

1. *WHO Expert Committee on Rabies, 8th report.* WHO Technical Report Series, No. 824. Geneva, Switzerland, World Health Organization, 1992, p 41.
2. Tizard I: Use of serologic testing to assess immune status of companion animals. *JAVMA* 213(1):54–60, 1998.
3. Aubert MF: Can vaccination validated by the titration of rabies antibodies in serum of cats and dogs be an alternative to quarantine measures? *Bureau Hyg Trop Med* 68(6):R2–R22, 1993.
4. Briggs DJ: Kansas State University Rabies Laboratory. Unpublished data from laboratory submissions, 1998.
5. Anonymous: Rabies, in: *OIE Manual of Standards for Diagnostic Tests and Vaccines*, 3rd ed. Paris, Office International des Epizooties, 1996, pp 211–213.
6. Briggs DJ, Smith JS, Mueller FL, et al: A comparison of two serological methods for detecting the immune response after rabies vaccination in dogs and cats being exported to rabies-free areas. *Biologicals*, in press.

Compendium of Animal Rabies Control, 1999*
National Association of State Public Health Veterinarians, Inc.

The purpose of this Compendium is to provide rabies information to veterinarians, public health officials, and others concerned with rabies control. These recommendations serve as the basis for animal rabies control programs throughout the United States and facilitate standardization of procedures among jurisdictions, thereby contributing to an effective national rabies control program. This document is reviewed annually and revised as necessary. Immunization procedure recommendations are contained in Part I; all animal rabies vaccines licensed by the United States Department of Agriculture (USDA) and marketed in the United States are listed in Part II; Part III details the principles of rabies control.

Part I: Recommendations for Parenteral Immunization Procedures

A. VACCINE ADMINISTRATION: All animal rabies vaccines should be restricted to use by, or under the direct supervision of, a veterinarian.

B. VACCINE SELECTION: In comprehensive rabies control programs, only vaccines with a 3-year duration of immunity should be used. This constitutes the most effective method of increasing the proportion of immunized dogs and cats in any population. (See Part II.)

C. ROUTE OF INOCULATION: All vaccines must be administered in accordance with the specifications of the product label or package insert. If administered intramuscularly, it must be at one site in the thigh.

D. WILDLIFE AND HYBRID ANIMAL VACCINATION: The efficacy of parenteral rabies vaccination of wildlife and hybrids (the offspring of wild animals crossbred to domestic dogs and cats) has not been established, and no such vaccine is licensed for these animals. Zoos or research institutions may establish vaccination programs which attempt to protect valuable animals, but these should not replace appropriate public health activities that protect humans.

E. ACCIDENTAL HUMAN EXPOSURE TO VACCINE: Accidental inoculation may occur during administration of animal rabies vaccine. Such exposure to inactivated vaccines constitutes no rabies hazard.

F. IDENTIFICATION OF VACCINATED ANIMALS: All agencies and veterinarians should adopt the standard tag system. This practice will aid the administration of local, state, national, and international control procedures. Animal license tags should be distinguishable in shape and color from rabies tags. Anodized aluminum rabies tags should be no less than 0.064 inches in thickness.

1. RABIES TAGS

YEAR	COLOR	SHAPE
1999	Green	Bell
2000	Red	Heart
2001	Blue	Rosette
2002	Orange	Oval

2. RABIES CERTIFICATE: All agencies and veterinarians should use the NASPHV form #51, "Rabies Vaccination Certificate," which can be obtained from vaccine manufacturers. Computer-generated forms containing the same information are acceptable.

THE NASPHV COMMITTEE
Suzanne R. Jenkins, VMD, MPH, Chair
Michael Auslander, DVM, MSPH
Robert H. Johnson, DVM
Mira J. Leslie, DVM
F. T. Satalowich, DVM, MSPH
Faye E. Sorhage, VMD, MPH

*Address all correspondence to:
Suzanne R. Jenkins, VMD, MPH
Virginia Department of Health
Office of Epidemiology
Post Office Box 2448, Room 113
Richmond, VA 23218

CONSULTANTS TO THE COMMITTEE
Deborah J. Briggs, PhD; Kansas State University Rabies
     Laboratory
James E. Childs, ScD; Centers for Disease Control
     and Prevention (CDC)
Mary Currier, MD, MPH; CSTE
David W. Dreesen, DVM, MPVM; private consultant
Nancy Frank, DVM, MPH; AVMA Council on Public Health and
     Regulatory Veterinary Medicine
Jim McCord, DVM; Animal Health Institute
Robert B. Miller, DVM, MPH; Animal and Plant Health
     Inspection Service, USDA
Charles E. Rupprecht, VMD, PhD; CDC
Charles V. Trimarchi, MS; New York State Rabies Laboratory

ENDORSED BY:
American Veterinary Medical Association (AVMA)
Council of State and Territorial Epidemiologists (CSTE)

Part II: Rabies Vaccines Licensed in U.S. and NASPHV Recommendations, 1999

Product Name	Produced by	Marketed by	For Use in	Dosage	Age at Primary Vaccination[1]	Booster Recommended	Route of Inoculation
A) MONOVALENT (inactivated)							
TRIMUNE	Fort Dodge Animal Health License No. 112	Fort Dodge Animal Health	Dogs Cats	1 ml 1 ml	3 months & 1 year later 3 months & 1 year later	Triennially Triennially	IM[2] IM
ANNUMUNE	Fort Dodge Animal Health License No. 112	Fort Dodge Animal Health	Dogs Cats	1 ml 1 ml	3 months 3 months	Annually Annually	IM IM
DEFENSOR 1	Pfizer, Incorporated License No. 189	Pfizer, Incorporated	Dogs Cats	1 ml 1 ml	3 months 3 months	Annually Annually	IM or SC[3] SC
DEFENSOR 3	Pfizer, Incorporated License No. 189	Pfizer, Incorporated	Dogs Cats Sheep Cattle	1 ml 1 ml 2 ml 2 ml	3 months & 1 year later 3 months & 1 year later 3 months 3 months	Triennially Triennially Annually Annually	IM or SC SC IM IM
RABDOMUN	Pfizer, Incorporated License No. 189	Schering-Plough	Dogs Cats Sheep Cattle	1 ml 1 ml 2 ml 2 ml	3 months & 1 year later 3 months & 1 year later 3 months 3 months	Triennially Triennially Annually Annually	IM or SC SC IM IM
RABDOMUN 1	Pfizer, Incorporated License No. 189	Schering-Plough	Dogs Cats	1 ml 1 ml	3 months 3 months	Annually Annually	IM or SC SC
RABVAC 1	Fort Dodge Animal Health License No. 112	Fort Dodge Animal Health	Dogs Cats	1 ml 1 ml	3 months 3 months	Annually Annually	IM or SC IM or SC
RABVAC 3	Fort Dodge Animal Health License No. 112	Fort Dodge Animal Health	Dogs Cats Horses	1 ml 1 ml 2 ml	3 months & 1 year later 3 months & 1 year later 3 months	Triennially Triennially Annually	IM or SC IM or SC IM
PRORAB-1	Intervet, Incorporated License No. 286	Intervet, Incorporated	Dogs Cats Sheep	1 ml 1 ml 2 ml	3 months 3 months 3 months	Annually Annually Annually	IM or SC IM or SC IM
PRORAB-3F	Intervet, Incorporated License No. 286	Intervet, Incorporated	Cats	1 ml	3 months & 1 year later	Triennially	IM or SC
IMRAB 3	Merial License No. 298	Merial	Dogs Cats Sheep Cattle Horses Ferrets	1 ml 1 ml 2 ml 2 ml 2 ml 1 ml	3 months & 1 year later 3 months & 1 year later 3 months & 1 year later 3 months 3 months 3 months	Triennially Triennially Triennially Annually Annually Annually	IM or SC IM or SC IM or SC IM or SC IM or SC SC
IMRAB BOVINE PLUS	Merial License No. 298	Merial	Cattle Horses Sheep	2 ml 2 ml 2 ml	3 months 3 months 3 months & 1 year later	Annually Annually Triennially	IM or SC IM or SC IM or SC
IMRAB 1	Merial License No. 298	Merial	Dogs Cats	1 ml 1 ml	3 months 3 months	Annually Annually	IM or SC IM or SC
IMRAB PUPPY[4]	Merial License No. 298	Merial	Dogs	1 ml	8 weeks & 1 year later	Annually	SC
B) COMBINATION (inactivated rabies)							
ECLIPSE 3 + FeLV/R	Fort Dodge Animal Health License No. 112	Schering-Plough	Cats	1 ml	3 months	Annually	IM or SC
ECLIPSE 4 + FeLV/R	Fort Dodge Animal Health License No. 112	Schering-Plough	Cats	1 ml	3 months	Annually	IM or SC
Fel-O-Guard 3 + FeLV/R	Fort Dodge Animal Health License No. 112	Fort Dodge Animal Health	Cats	1 ml	3 months	Annually	IM or SC
Fel-O-Guard 4 + FeLV/R	Fort Dodge Animal Health License No. 112	Fort Dodge Animal Health	Cats	1 ml	3 months	Annually	IM or SC
Fel-O-Vax PCT-R	Fort Dodge Animal Health License No. 112	Fort Dodge Animal Health	Cats	1 ml	3 months & 1 year later	Triennially	IM
FELINE 4 + IMRAB	Merial License No. 298	Merial	Cats	1 ml	3 months & 1 year later	Triennially	SC
FELINE 3 + IMRAB	Merial License No. 298	Merial	Cats	1 ml	3 months & 1 year later	Triennially	SC
PUREVAX Feline 4/ Rabies + LEUCAT	Merial License No. 298	Merial	Cats	1 ml	8 weeks & 1 year later	Annually	SC
PUREVAX Feline 4/ Rabies	Merial License No. 298	Merial	Cats	1 ml	8 weeks & 1 year later	Annually	SC
PUREVAX Feline 3/ Rabies + LEUCAT	Merial License No. 298	Merial	Cats	1 ml	8 weeks & 1 year later	Annually	SC

1 Three months of age (or older) and revaccinated one year later.
2 Intramuscularly.
3 Subcutaneously.
4 Marketed in combination packages only.

Product Name	Produced by	Marketed by	For Use in	Dosage	Age at Primary Vaccination[1]	Booster Recommended	Route of Inoculation
PUREVAX Feline 3/ Rabies	Merial License No. 298	Merial	Cats	1 ml	8 weeks & 1 year later	Annually	SC
PUREVAX Feline Rabies	Merial License No. 298	Merial	Cats	1 ml	8 weeks & 1 year later	Annually	SC
EQUINE POTOMAVAC + IMRAB	Merial License No. 298	Merial	Horses	1 ml	3 months	Annually	IM
MYSTIQUE II	Bayer Corporation License No. 52	Bayer Corporation	Horses	1 ml	3 months	Annually	IM
RECOMBITEK C4 + IMRAB PUPPY	Merial License No. 298	Merial	Dogs	1 ml	8 weeks & 1 year later	Annually	SC
RECOMBITEK C4/CV + IMRAB PUPPY	Merial License No. 298	Merial	Dogs	1 ml	8 weeks & 1 year later	Annually	SC
C) ORAL (rabies glycoprotein, live vaccinia vector) - RESTRICTED TO USE IN STATE AND FEDERAL RABIES CONTROL PROGRAMS							
RABORAL V-RG	Merial License No. 298	Merial	Raccoons	N/A	N/A	Determined by state authorities	Oral

Part III: Rabies Control

A. PRINCIPLES OF RABIES CONTROL

1. **RABIES EXPOSURE:** Rabies is transmitted only when the virus is introduced into bite wounds, open cuts in skin, or onto mucous membranes.

2. **HUMAN RABIES PREVENTION:** Rabies in humans can be prevented either by eliminating exposures to rabid animals or by providing exposed persons with prompt local treatment of wounds combined with appropriate passive and active immunization. The rationale for recommending preexposure and postexposure rabies prophylaxis and details of their administration can be found in the current recommendations of the Immunization Practices Advisory Committee (ACIP) of the Public Health Service (PHS). These recommendations, along with information concerning the current local and regional status of animal rabies and the availability of human rabies biologics, are available from state health departments.

3. **DOMESTIC ANIMALS:** Local governments should initiate and maintain effective programs to ensure vaccination of all dogs, cats, and ferrets and to remove strays and unwanted animals. Such procedures in the United States have reduced laboratory confirmed cases in dogs from 6,949 in 1947 to 126 in 1997. Since more rabies cases are reported annually involving cats (300 in 1997) than dogs, vaccination of cats should be required. The recommended vaccination procedures and the licensed animal vaccines are specified in Parts I and II of the Compendium.

4. **RABIES IN WILDLIFE:** The control of rabies among wildlife reservoirs is difficult. Vaccination of free-ranging wildlife or selective population reduction may be useful in some situations, but the success of such procedures depends on the circumstances surrounding each rabies outbreak. (See Part C. Control Methods in Wildlife.)

B. CONTROL METHODS IN DOMESTIC AND CONFINED ANIMALS

1. **PREEXPOSURE VACCINATION AND MANAGEMENT**
   Parenteral animal rabies vaccines should be administered only by, or under the direct supervision of, a veterinarian. This is the only way to ensure that a responsible person can be held accountable to assure the public that the animal has been properly vaccinated. Within 1 month after primary vaccination, a peak rabies antibody titer is reached and the animal can be considered immunized. An animal is currently vaccinated and is considered immunized if it was vaccinated at least 30 days previously, and all vaccinations have been administered in accordance with this Compendium. Regardless of the age at initial vaccination, a second vaccination should be given one year later. (See Parts I and II for recommended vaccines and procedures.)

   (a) DOGS, CATS, AND FERRETS
   All dogs, cats, and ferrets should be vaccinated against rabies at 3 months of age and revaccinated in accordance with Part II of this Compendium. If a previously vaccinated animal is overdue for a booster, it should be revaccinated with a single dose of vaccine and placed on an annual or triennial schedule depending on the type of vaccine used.

   (b) LIVESTOCK
   It is neither economically feasible nor justified from a public health standpoint to vaccinate all livestock against rabies. However, consideration should be given to vaccination of livestock which are particularly valuable and/or may have frequent contact with humans.

(c) OTHER ANIMALS
  (1) WILD
      No parenteral rabies vaccine is licensed for use in wild animals. Because of the risk of rabies in wild animals (especially raccoons, skunks, coyotes, foxes, and bats), the AVMA, the NASPHV, and the CSTE strongly recommend the enactment of state laws prohibiting the importation, distribution, relocation, or keeping of wild animals or hybrids as pets.

  (2) MAINTAINED IN EXHIBITS AND IN ZOOLOGICAL PARKS
      Captive animals not completely excluded from all contact with rabies vectors can become infected. Moreover, wild animals may be incubating rabies when initially captured; therefore, wild-caught animals susceptible to rabies should be quarantined for a minimum of 180 days before exhibition. Employees who work with animals at such facilities should receive preexposure rabies immunization. The use of pre- or postexposure rabies immunizations of employees who work with animals at such facilities may reduce the need for euthanasia of captive animals.

2. **STRAY ANIMALS**
   Stray dogs, cats, or ferrets should be removed from the community. Local health departments and animal control officials can enforce the removal of strays more effectively if owned animals are confined or kept on leash. Strays should be impounded for at least 3 days to give owners sufficient time to reclaim animals and to determine if human exposure has occurred.

3. **IMPORTATION AND INTERSTATE MOVEMENT OF ANIMALS**
   (a) INTERNATIONAL
       CDC regulates the importation of dogs and cats into the United States, but present PHS regulations (42 CFR No. 71.51) governing the importation of such animals are insufficient to prevent the introduction of rabid animals into the country. All dogs and cats imported from countries with endemic rabies should be currently vaccinated against rabies as recommended in this Compendium. The appropriate public health official of the state of destination should be notified within 72 hours of any unvaccinated dog or cat imported into his or her jurisdiction. The conditional admission of such animals into the United States is subject to state and local laws governing rabies. Failure to comply with these requirements should be promptly reported to the Division of Quarantine, CDC, 404-639-8107.

   (b) INTERSTATE
       Prior to interstate movement, dogs, cats, and ferrets should be currently vaccinated against rabies in accordance with the Compendium's recommendations (See Part III, B.1. Preexposure Vaccination and Management). Animals in transit should be accompanied by a currently valid NASPHV Form #51, Rabies Vaccination Certificate.

4. **ADJUNCT PROCEDURES**
   Methods or procedures which enhance rabies control include:
   (a) LICENSURE. Registration or licensure of all dogs, cats, and ferrets may be used to aid in rabies control. A fee is frequently charged for such licensure and revenues collected are used to maintain rabies or animal control programs. Vaccination is an essential prerequisite to licensure.

   (b) CANVASSING OF AREA. House-to-house canvassing by animal control personnel facilitates enforcement of vaccination and licensure requirements.

   (c) CITATIONS. Citations are legal summonses issued to owners for violations, including the failure to vaccinate or license their animals. The authority for officers to issue citations should be an integral part of each animal control program.

   (d) ANIMAL CONTROL. All communities should incorporate stray animal control, leash laws, and training of personnel in their programs.

5. **POSTEXPOSURE MANAGEMENT**
   ANY ANIMAL POTENTIALLY EXPOSED TO RABIES VIRUS (See Part III, A. 1. Rabies Exposure) BY A WILD, CARNIVOROUS MAMMAL OR A BAT THAT IS NOT AVAILABLE FOR TESTING SHOULD BE REGARDED AS HAVING BEEN EXPOSED TO RABIES.

   (a) DOGS, CATS, AND FERRETS
       Unvaccinated dogs, cats, and ferrets exposed to a rabid animal should be euthanized immediately. If the owner is unwilling to have this done, the animal should be placed in strict isolation for 6 months and vaccinated 1 month before being released. Animals with expired vaccinations need to be evaluated on a case by case basis. Dogs, cats, and ferrets that are currently vaccinated should be revaccinated immediately, kept under the owner's control, and observed for 45 days.

(b) LIVESTOCK

All species of livestock are susceptible to rabies; cattle and horses are among the most frequently infected. Livestock exposed to a rabid animal and currently vaccinated with a vaccine approved by USDA for that species should be re-vaccinated immediately and observed for 45 days. Unvaccinated livestock should be slaughtered immediately. If the owner is unwilling to have this done, the animal should be kept under very close observation for 6 months.

The following are recommendations for owners of unvaccinated livestock exposed to rabid animals:

(1) If the animal is slaughtered within 7 days of being bitten, its tissues may be eaten without risk of infection, provided liberal portions of the exposed area are discarded. Federal meat inspectors must reject for slaughter any animal known to have been exposed to rabies within 8 months.

(2) Neither tissues nor milk from a rabid animal should be used for human or animal consumption. However, since pasteurization temperatures will inactivate rabies virus, drinking pasteurized milk or eating cooked meat does not constitute a rabies exposure.

(3) It is rare to have more than one rabid animal in a herd, or herbivore to herbivore transmission; therefore, it may not be necessary to restrict the rest of the herd if a single animal has been exposed to or infected by rabies.

(c) OTHER ANIMALS

Other animals bitten by a rabid animal should be euthanized immediately. Animals maintained in USDA licensed research facilities or accredited zoological parks should be evaluated on a case by case basis.

6. MANAGEMENT OF ANIMALS THAT BITE HUMANS

A healthy dog, cat, or ferret that bites a person should be confined and observed for 10 days; it is recommended that rabies vaccine not be administered during the observation period. Such animals should be evaluated by a veterinarian at the first sign of illness during confinement. Any illness in the animal should be reported immediately to the local health department. If signs suggestive of rabies develop, the animal should be euthanized, its head removed, and the head shipped under refrigeration (not frozen) for examination of the brain by a qualified laboratory designated by the local or state health department. Any stray or unwanted dog, cat, or ferret that bites a person may be euthanized immediately and the head submitted as described above for rabies examination. Other biting animals which might have exposed a person to rabies should be reported immediately to the local health department. Prior vaccination of an animal may not preclude the necessity for euthanasia and testing if the period of virus shedding is unknown for that species. Management of animals other than dogs, cats, and ferrets depends on the species, the circumstances of the bite, the epidemiology of rabies in the area, and the biting animal's history, current health status, and potential for exposure to rabies.

C. CONTROL METHODS IN WILDLIFE

The public should be warned not to handle wildlife. Wild mammals and hybrids that bite or otherwise expose people, pets or livestock should be considered for euthanasia and rabies examination. A person bitten by any wild mammal should immediately report the incident to a physician who can evaluate the need for antirabies treatment. (See current rabies prophylaxis recommendations of the ACIP.)

1. TERRESTRIAL MAMMALS

The use of licensed oral vaccines for the mass immunization of free-ranging wildlife should be considered in selected situations, with the approval of the state agency responsible for animal rabies control. Continuous and persistent government-funded programs for trapping or poisoning wildlife are not cost effective in reducing wildlife rabies reservoirs on a statewide basis. However, limited control in high-contact areas (picnic grounds, camps, suburban areas) may be indicated for the removal of selected high-risk species of wildlife. The state wildlife agency and state health department should be consulted for coordination of any proposed vaccination or population reduction programs.

2. BATS

(a) Indigenous rabid bats have been reported from every state except Hawaii, and have caused rabies in at least 32 humans in the United States. It is neither feasible nor desirable, however, to control rabies in bats by programs to reduce bat populations.

(b) Bats should be excluded from houses and adjacent structures to prevent direct association with humans. Such structures should then be made bat-proof by sealing entrances used by bats.

State and local requirements vary about reporting animal bites. Check with local authorities on local rules and requirements. This worksheet will help you in the reporting process.

RABIES CASE INVESTIGATION WORKSHEET

A. Complete this section for potential human exposures to rabies

Name: _____

Age: _____ Sex: _____

Did the victim previously complete a series of rabies vaccine?
☐ Yes ☐ No

Has the victim had a tetanus vaccine within the past 5 years?
☐ Yes ☐ No
If no, tetanus vaccine is needed.

Type of exposure (e.g., bite, scratch): _____
Anatomic site: _____
Exposure date: _____

Describe events that led to exposure:
_____
_____
_____

B. Complete this section for potential animal exposures to rabies

How many animals exposed? _____

Date of exposure: _____

List each animal separately:
Species	Proof of current rabies immunization
_____	☐ Yes ☐ No
_____	☐ Yes ☐ No
_____	☐ Yes ☐ No

Veterinarian's name: _____

Telephone number: _____

Describe events that led to exposure:
_____
_____
_____

C. Complete this section for the animal(s) causing the exposure

Number of animals causing exposure? _____

List each animal separately:

Species	Proof of current rabies vaccination	Animal confined?
_____	☐ Yes ☐ No	☐ Yes ☐ No
_____	☐ Yes ☐ No	☐ Yes ☐ No
_____	☐ Yes ☐ No	☐ Yes ☐ No

D. Complete this section for the person or animal identified in A or B above

Has the person or animal been potentially exposed to rabies? ☐ Yes ☐ No
If yes, complete Sections E and (F or G)

E. Disposition of animal causing exposure

Check one:
☐ Dog or cat confined for 10 days
  Start date: _____ End date: _____
  Location of confinement: _____

☐ Animal sacrificed and tested for rabies
  Test result: _____
☐ Other: _____

F. Complete this section for exposed humans

Check one:
☐ Person received HRIG and 5 doses of rabies vaccine
☐ Person started series but did not complete series because:
  ☐ Animal was not rabid
  ☐ Patient refused further treatment
  ☐ Patient was lost to follow-up
☐ Person refused treatment
☐ Other: _____

G. Complete this section for exposed animals

Check one:
☐ Animal was sacrificed. Date: _____
☐ Animal was revaccinated and observed for 45 days
☐ Animal was revaccinated and observed for 90 days
☐ Animal was quarantined for 6 months then vaccinated 1 month before release
☐ Animal was quarantined for 6 months
☐ Other: _____

Notes: _____
_____
_____

Name of person doing investigation: _____

Date: _____

MERIAL

Source: Kansas Department of Health and Environment.

Continuing Education Test (Answer Form on p. 87)

1. **Rabies in the United States is maintained by several terrestrial reservoir species, including the:**
   a. Skunk, rabbit, and bat.
   b. Raccoon, skunk, and coyote.
   c. Horse, dog, and bat.
   d. Coyote, mongoose, and gray fox.

2. **Control of wildlife-mediated rabies in some countries is carried out by:**
   a. Programs of oral vaccination of wildlife.
   b. Programs to vaccinate people at risk of exposure to wildlife.
   c. Programs to trap animals, vaccinate them, and release them back to the wild.
   d. None of the above.

3. **The most common method of transmission of the rabies virus is:**
   a. Consumption of rabies-infected animals.
   b. Bite or scratch wounds inflicted by infected animals.
   c. Airborne transmission of viral particles.
   d. Transplacentally to the infected animals' offspring.

4. **One explanation for the prolonged incubation period of rabies is:**
   a. The virus becomes dormant within nerve tissue.
   b. An amplification step occurs within myocytes before infection of peripheral nerves takes place.
   c. The virus needs specific cellular nutrients to survive and will encapsulate until they are present.
   d. All of the above.

5. **Dogs that bite humans are often quarantined for 10 days because:**
   a. The incubation period of rabies in dogs is less than 10 days.
   b. Virus will be shed in an infected dog's saliva for only a few days before the onset of clinical signs.
   c. If the dog is healthy after 10 days, it has not been exposed to the rabies virus.
   d. a and c.

6. **In the United States, feline rabies cases:**
   a. Occur most commonly in geographic areas experiencing epizootics of rabies in raccoons.
   b. Have caused several states to pass laws to make rabies vaccination of cats mandatory.
   c. Have surpassed those in dogs since 1981.
   d. All of the above.

7. **Rabies vaccination of horses:**
   a. Is not recommended unless other horses in the area have been diagnosed with rabies.
   b. Should be given prophylactically if a horse is presented with neurologic signs.
   c. Is required in the United States to transport a horse across state lines.
   d. May help establish an immune barrier between humans and the wildlife population.

8. **When a person is bitten by a mouse:**
   a. Postexposure prophylaxis is not usually recommended because the risk of rabies is low.
   b. Postexposure prophylaxis is administered if the animal is not available for testing.
   c. A health official may recommend testing of the mouse for rabies if it was sick or acting strangely.
   d. a and c.

9. **The incubation period for rabies in humans:**
   a. Is usually less than 10 days.
   b. Has been reported to be as long as 6 years.
   c. Is dependent on factors such as the site of inoculation and the dose of rabies virus.
   d. b and c.

10. **Epidemiologic evidence shows that:**
    a. Routine rabies vaccination of dogs has no effect on the rabies death rate in people that have been bitten by dogs.
    b. Routine rabies vaccination of dogs, along with animal control programs, decreases the number of rabies deaths in people that have been bitten by dogs.
    c. Feline rabies cases in the United States have been declining for the last 20 years.
    d. None of the above.

11. **Currently, licensed animal rabies vaccines:**
    a. Must protect at least 90% of the vaccinates against challenge infection.
    b. Are tested by evaluation of antibody titer rather than by challenge tests.
    c. Are not approved for use in ferrets.
    d. None of the above.

12. **Upon exposure to rabies, a person that has received rabies preexposure immunization:**
    a. Will not need as lengthy postexposure treatment as a person with no immunization history.
    b. Needs to be given human rabies immune globulin (HRIG) but requires no other treatment.
    c. Should be started on preexposure prophylaxis only if antibody is not detected in a serum sample taken at the time of exposure.
    d. a and c.

13. **It is very likely that rabies will remain a major public health issue because:**
    a. Wildlife epizootics will continue to expand.
    b. New rabies viral variants such as the one recently found in bats are being identified.
    c. The cost associated with rabies control and prevention is increasing.
    d. All of the above.

14. **If the entire head of a suspected rabid animal is sent to the diagnostic laboratory:**
    a. The head should be frozen immediately after collection.
    b. The head should be refrigerated until it arrives at the laboratory.
    c. No method of preservative should be used because this will interfere with reliable diagnosis.
    d. It should be placed in formalin.

15. **The standard and preferred test for the diagnosis of rabies is:**
    a. Identification of Negri bodies within the Purkinje cells of the cerebellum and in the pyramidal cells of the hippocampus.
    b. Fluorescent antibody test for virus.
    c. Growing the virus in cell culture and inoculating mice.
    d. Enzyme-linked immunosorbent assay of serum.

16. **Sensitive diagnosis of rabies by immunofluorescence is hampered by:**
    a. Poor-quality samples.
    b. Brain tissue that has been formalin fixed.
    c. Repeated freeze-thaw cycles of samples.
    d. All of the above.

17. **Recombinant rabies vaccines:**
    a. Have been used successfully in wildlife vaccination programs.
    b. Invoke a protective immune response when administered orally, subcutaneously, or intramuscularly.
    c. Utilize a glycoprotein from the outer surface of the rabies virus.
    d. All of the above.

18. **Research indicates that puppies with maternal antibodies against rabies:**
    a. Should not be vaccinated against rabies until they are more than 4 months old.
    b. Respond to rabies immunization as young as 6 weeks of age.
    c. Are protected against natural infection until they are 6 months old.
    d. None of the above.

19. **The governments of many rabies-free areas are reevaluating their quarantine systems because:**
    a. It is currently recognized that the incubation period of rabies is less than 3 months.
    b. Our mobile society has exerted public pressure.
    c. Vaccines are 100% effective; therefore, quarantine is not needed in vaccinated animals.
    d. Domesticated pets are not a threat to rabies-free areas.

20. **The requirements for dogs and cats entering a rabies-free area can generally be obtained from:**
    a. The airline that will be used to transport the animal.
    b. The country's department of agriculture.
    c. The country's governmental consulate in Washington, DC.
    d. b and c.

Answer Form

Circle the best answer for each question:

1	2	3	4	5	6	7	8	9	10
A	A	A	A	A	A	A	A	A	A
B	B	B	B	B	B	B	B	B	B
C	C	C	C	C	C	C	C	C	C
D	D	D	D	D	D	D	D	D	D

11	12	13	14	15	16	17	18	19	20
A	A	A	A	A	A	A	A	A	A
B	B	B	B	B	B	B	B	B	B
C	C	C	C	C	C	C	C	C	C
D	D	D	D	D	D	D	D	D	D

Fill out answer form, provide information requested on opposite side of form, and submit this sheet with a check for $30 (payable to Regents of the University of California) by November 1, 2000, to:

Donald J. Klingborg, DVM
Office of Public Programs
School of Veterinary Medicine
1 Shields Avenue
University of California–Davis
Davis, CA 95616

Rabies: Guidelines for Medical Professionals
Sponsored by Merial

How to Document Your Continuing Education

This monograph is approved for 2 hours of continuing education credit by The University of California–Davis School of Veterinary Medicine. Readers should consult their state licensing authority regarding acceptability of credit.

A fee of $30 covers registration, test scoring, and individual notification of results. Payment must accompany each answer sheet submitted.

For more information, contact Donald J. Klingborg, DVM, at the Office of Public Programs, School of Veterinary Medicine, 1 Shields Ave., University of California–Davis, Davis, California 95616 or by phone at 530-752-1524.

NOTE: Photocopies of the answer form may be submitted for continuing education credit. The $30 registration fee must accompany each form or photocopy submitted. Be sure to photocopy and complete both sides of this form for each submission.

Name: _____

                           Last   First   Middle Initial

SS #: _____ – _____ – _____

Telephone: _____

Practice Name: _____

Practice Address: _____

City: _____ State: _____ Zip: _____